LEARNING MATERIALS
ON
MENTAL HEALTH

An Introduction

The University of Manchester

Department of Health

British Library Cataloguing in Publication Data. A catalogue record for this book is available from the British Library.
ISBN 0906 107 71 7

Complementary title available from The University of Manchester "Learning Materials on Mental Health Risk Assessment."

Both publications available from:
The School of Psychiatry and Behavioural Sciences
Mathematics Building
The Unversity of Manchester
Oxford Road
Manchester M13 9PL
Telephone: 0161-275 5221

EDITORS

Mrs. Heather Bagley (Project Manager)
Ms. Barbara Hatfield
Professor Peter Huxley

AUTHORS

Ms. Corinna Alberg
Research Associate,
The University of Manchester

Mrs. Heather Bagley
Research Associate,
The University of Manchester

Dr. Leonard Bowers
*Coordinator of the Psychiatric Nursing
Research and Development Unit,*
Manchester Metropolitan University
and Tameside and Glossop CPS NHS
Trust

Professor Alistair Burns
Professor of Old Age Psychiatry,
The University of Manchester

Professor David Challis
*Professor of Psychiatric Social Work
and Community Care,*
The University of Manchester

Ms. Barbara Hatfield
Lecturer in Psychiatric Social Work,
The University of Manchester

Professor Peter Huxley
Professor of Psychiatric Social Work,
The University of Manchester

Professor Michael Kerfoot
*School of Psychiatary
and Behavioural Sciences,*
The University of Manchester

Professor Shon Lewis
Professor of Psychiatry,
The University of Manchester

Ms. Dorothy Lott
*Team Leader, Mental Health Support
Team for Homeless People, Hostels
Liaison Group,*
Nottingham.

Ms. Branwen McHugh
*Therapist, Child and Adolescent
Psychiatry, Carol Kendrick Unit,*
Duchess of York Hospital, Withington,
Greater Manchester.

Mr. Brian Minty
Lecturer in Psychiatric Social Work
The University of Manchester

Mr. Steven Moss
*Senior Research Fellow,
Hester Adrian Research Centre,*
The University of Manchester

Mr. David Sawdon
Independent Training Consultant,
Barnsley

Ms. Catherine Sawdon
Independent Training Consultant,
Barnsley

Ms. Jeni Webster
Lecturer in Psychiatric Social Work,
The University of Manchester

STEERING GROUP MEMBERS

The work was commissioned by the Department of Health and supported by the Steering Group. Their help throughout the development and production of the materials is gratefully acknowledged.

Professor Louis Appleby
*School of Psychiatary
and Behavioural Sciences,*
The University of Manchester

Mrs. Heather Bagley
Research Associate,
The University of Manchester

Ms. Reba Bhaduri
Social Services Inspector,
Department of Health

Mr. Michael Dewane
Social Services Inspector,
Department of Health

Mr. Tom Foster
*Ex-director of
Lancashire Social Services*

Ms. Jean Garlic
Support Services Manager,
Making Space, Warrington

Ms. Barbara Hatfield
Lecturer in Psychiatric Social Work,
The University of Manchester

Mr. Michael Hennessey
Director of Social Services, Shropshire

Mr. David Horsler
Training Officer,
Salford Social Services

Professor Peter Huxley
Professor of Psychiatric Social Work,
The University of Manchester

Mr. Harrie Kandola
*Publications Designer,
International and
Public Relations Office,*
The University of Manchester

Ms. Andrea Leonard
Manager, NHS Executive,
Mental Health and
Community Care Division

Mr. Nick Metcalfe
Officer in Charge,
Daisy Bank Day Centre, Manchester

Mr. Barry Norman
Social Service Inspector,
Department of Health

Mr. David Pottage
*Research Fellow in
Psychiatric Social Work,*
The University of Manchester

Ms. Melissa Wallder
Executive Officer, NHS Executive,
Mental Health and
Community Care Division

ACKNOWLEDGEMENTS

We are grateful to the following people and organisations for their assistance
in preparing and commenting on materials.

Professor Louis Appleby
School of Psychiatry
and Behavioural Sciences,
The University of Manchester

Dr. Linda Gask
Senior Lecturer in Psychiatry,
National Primary Care Research and
Development Centre,
The University of Manchester

Ms. Helen Sumner
Principal Officer, Adult Services,
Cheshire County Council, Social
Services Group.

Ms. Melba Wilson
Researcher and Writer, formerly with
the NHS Mental Health Task Force's
Regional Race Programme

Ms. Jennifer Barnard
Director of Social Services,
Newcastle Upon Tyne Social Services
Department and Chair, ADSS Mental
Health Strategy Group.

Mrs. Liz Potter
Senior Training Officer,
Wandsworth Social Services,
Department Training Section

Mrs. Barbara Robertson
Co-ordinator, Merseyside Family
Mediation Service, Liverpool

Mr. David Lee
Development Officer (Mental Health),
Trafford Social Services.

Ms. Gwen Ovshinsky
Service Planning Manager -
Mental Health,
Hertfordshire Social Services

Mr. Barry Windle
Mental Health Services Manager,
Rochdale Social Services.

Mr. Philip Radcliffe
Radcliffe Associates,
Whaley Bridge, Derbyshire.

**African-Caribbean Mental Health
Project**, Hulme, Manchester.

Bolton Social Services Department

Creative Support
Manchester.

Making Space
Warrington

**Manchester Social Services
Department**

**Rochdale Social Services
Department**

**Stockport Social Services
Department**

**Students of the 1995/6
Certificate In Mental Health Care**
The University of Manchester

**Tameside Social Services
Department**

Turning Point
Scotland

CONTENTS

INTRODUCTION

Who are the Training Materials for?

These materials are designed to help those who are, or may be, working with people experiencing mental health problems. The materials will be useful to mental health support workers, residential and day care workers, and to social workers whose training has not included a substantial mental health component.

What are the Training Materials about?

The materials are designed to provide you with up-to-date information on various aspects of mental health care. After working through the materials you should be better able to answer the following questions:

- What is a mental health problem and how can I recognise one?

- What should I do when I think a person might be mentally ill?

- How are services organised to help?

- Are there any special problems I should know about?

- How can I become informed about and make use of the perspective of the service users and their children and carers?

Content of the Modules

There are seven modules in this volume. Each module can stand alone or form part of a wider training programme.

- **Module 1** - We focus on the recognition of mental health problems. We aim to answer such questions as: Who is more likely to develop a mental health problem? How common is it? How long will it last?

- **Module 2** - Our aim is to identify the major interventions and treatments currently available from hospital and community mental health services. We provide information on a multi-disciplinary approach to mental health care and demonstrate the various routes of referral for specialised help.

- **Module 3** - We aim to present the learner with an up-to-date summary of the legislation and guidance relevant to mental health care. The Care Programme Approach, care management and the *1983, Mental Health Act*, are described, together with other relevant provisions.

- **Module 4** - We aim to outline issues relating to client groups which pose particular challenges to the learner. Addressed issues include: gender, race and culture, learning disability, and young and older people with mental health problems.

- **Module 5** - We focus on special issues relating to people with mental health problems. Homelessness, risk of violence, suicide and substance misuse are described.

- **Module 6** - Our aim is to demonstrate the importance of the user perspective (how the user sees his/her difficulties). We also focus on the impact of mental illness on the families of people with mental health problems, examining the consequences of the caring role. We highlight the problems experienced by children with parents experiencing mental health difficulties.

- **Module 7** - This final module will provide sample training exercises that can be used with the pack. We see them as examples of the types of exercises that trainers in the field may like to develop in conjunction with the six preceding modules.

How can the materials be used?

The material is in a number of modules and how you choose to use them is up to you. You may be interested in reading a particular module or may want to work your way through the entire package. The materials can be used on a self-learning basis or for group learning. Some group training exercises are given as an example of the types of activities that can be undertaken. Also, within each module, we have provided "dilemmas" and "activities" which we hope will both stimulate discussion with other professionals and encourage you to think about how the issues raised in the materials might relate to your place of work.

The materials have been designed so that they can be photocopied easily. Contained within the "Trainers Appendix" are certain cases and major points taken from the main text of the modules. These have been set out in a style specifically designed for photocopying. No permission is required for photocopying the materials but the authors should be acknowledged.

All the names used in the case studies, examples, dilemmas and exercises are fictitious.

A sister set of materials is also available for professionals involved in assessing risk "Learning materials on Mental Health Risk Assessment". Whilst this is primarily designed to meet the learning needs of professionals specialising in mental health, some of the information provided may be of use to you.

module 1

RECOGNITION OF MENTAL HEALTH PROBLEMS

AIMS & OBJECTIVES

After you have worked through this module you should be better able to:

- Discuss what is meant by the terms "mental health" and "mental illness".

- Identify key symptoms associated with specific mental health problems.

- Discuss factors which have been identified as potential causes of mental illness.

- Discuss the prognosis of specific mental health problems.

MENTAL HEALTH & MENTAL HEALTH PROBLEMS

MODULE 1

WHAT DO "MENTAL HEALTH" AND "MENTAL ILLNESS" MEAN?

Jackie is seen dancing and singing with her friends in a pub one Friday evening.
Is Jackie mentally ill?

One morning, Jessica is seen dancing and singing whilst in the middle of the street. She was not under the influence of alcohol or drugs at the time.
Is Jessica mentally ill?

Mr. Bailey is so depressed following the death of his wife two days ago, that he feels life is no longer worth living. He has not slept well for the past two nights, is finding it difficult to eat and is quite clearly in utter despair.
Is Mr. Bailey mentally ill?

Mr. Choudrey's wife died seven years ago. Over the past three weeks he has become increasingly depressed. He is having problems sleeping and is losing weight because he cannot face his food.
Is Mr. Choudrey mentally ill?

The examples above demonstrate that "mental health" and "mental ill-health" are difficult to define. The circumstances in which a behaviour occurs are clearly important. In addition, if the behaviour is regarded as "understandable under the circumstances", then it is probably less likely to be considered "unhealthy".

It is not enough to say that mental health is "normality", as we each have different ideas of what is normal. What one person considers to be unusual, inappropriate or strange behaviour, may appear acceptable and understandable to another person. What we think of as normal depends on many things, such as past experiences, education, social expectations and cultural background.

There is no clear cut dividing line between health and ill-health. We all have periods of mental distress as we have periods of physical ill-health. Usually these periods are short and we recover without medical intervention. Some people, however, experience more frequent or severe periods of mental ill-health and a few have very long lasting problems.

Two questions help us recognise mental ill-health:

• Severity - Is the individual's suffering severe and distressing, beyond what he/she feels able to bear? It is, however, important to note that in some cases when someone is diagnosed as having a severe mental illness, the person may not realise that he/she is "suffering".

• Change/loss of function - Are the symptoms of the person's illness making it impossible for him or her to carry on as normal? In other words, is the condition clearly affecting how the person lives his or her life? These changes may be personal - for example, poor sleep, or social - inability to work or form relationships.

Attempts have been made to define mental illness - The World Health Organization has defined it as

"A term used by doctors and other health professionals to describe clinically recognisable patterns of psychological symptoms or behaviour causing acute or chronic ill-health, personal distress or distress to others." [1]

A doctor or a psychiatrist looks for certain signs and symptoms when deciding if someone is mentally ill. When a number of these occur together in a person, it is known as a syndrome. Whilst a social worker or support worker is not expected to diagnose mental illness, they must understand enough to be able to make an appropriate referral, or participate in the delivery of a care plan.

WHY DIAGNOSE OR CLASSIFY?

A diagnosis is important both for the person experiencing a mental health problem and for the health workers involved in planning care. The person who is distressed or disabled needs to make sense of the experience.

- **What is it?**
- **Why is this happening to me?**
- **What can be done to help me?**
- **Will I ever recover?**

A diagnosis may help to answer such questions and can sometimes make it easier for health professionals to develop a treatment plan.

Psychiatrists also classify mental illnesses as a way of trying to understand them. Classification brings together diagnoses that are related because they have similar symptoms, causes or treatments. The main classification system in use in the United Kingdom is known as ICD-10. This book contains information which psychiatrists use in classifying mental illnesses and disorders. It is important, too, to recognise the limitations of these "diagnostic classifications". On their own they are not particularly good indicators of the outcome of the illness nor of the costs of care to be provided.

There are also negative aspects to diagnoses. They can become labels, for example, "he's a schizophrenic", where the diagnosis is used to describe the person. This pigeon-holing effect can result in people being treated according to their label, rather than as individuals. In addition, people with diagnoses can begin to respond to the labels they have been given and behave as they believe they are expected to - the "sick role".

It is important to remember that many people recover from periods of mental illness, and re-establish their usual social roles.

WHAT TYPES OF MENTAL HEALTH PROBLEMS ARE THERE?

In classifying mental illnesses, two broad distinctions arise:

- The first point distinguishes **organic** and **functional** disorders. "Organic" means that there is a clear biological cause. An example of this is dementia.

"Functional" means that no definite biological cause has (yet) been found.

- The second distinction is between "neuroses" and "psychoses". The symptoms associated with neurotic disorders may be regarded as severe forms of normal experiences, such as depression or anxiety. Neurotic disorders include depressive illness, generalised anxiety disorder, phobia and panic disorder. Psychotic symptoms are different in that they are not common experiences. Many psychotic illnesses lead to hallucinations (the experience of a person sensing something that is not there - but which he/she experiences as real) and delusions (mistaken beliefs that are firmly held, in spite of logical arguments to the contrary). For example, a woman may believe that her neighbours are plotting against her and can hear her neighbours voices, even though they live at the other end of the street. Conditions which fall into the category of psychoses include schizophrenia and manic-depressive illness. (The above terms are explained later in this module).

The term "severe mental health problems" is sometimes used to refer to the psychoses. However, some people with neurotic conditions are no less disabled by their problem.

Another term commonly used is **personality disorder (PD)**, examples include "borderline PD" and "anti-social PD". Personality disorders are present throughout life and are diagnosed when patterns of thinking and behaviour, such as shyness, impulsive actions, or anti-social behaviours cause difficulties for a person. Some people believe that this category of mental disorders has been reserved for people whose diagnosis is uncertain or who are difficult to engage in treatment.

In this module we will look at the following conditions:

- **Schizophrenia**
- **Mood disorders -**
    - *Depression*
    - *Manic-depression (bi-polar disorder)*
- **Dementia**
- **Generalized anxiety disorder**
- **Phobias**
- **Panic disorder**
- **Personality disorders**

SCHIZOPHRENIA

CASE STUDY: Barry

Barry Horton is 25 years old and lives with his middle-aged-parents.

Last year, Barry began to become more and more withdrawn and his parents felt he was "strange". When they spoke to him, he did not reply properly, stared a lot, and seemed preoccupied with an inner world, often "talking to himself". One night he cut up several items of clothing and threw them out of his bedroom window. He then became "explosive", shouting and running outside for no clear reason. He said that voices told him he was smelling of urine, and he couldn't prove them wrong because "they come from another atmosphere".

Barry was hospitalised twice in the following year and treated with antipsychotic medication. This had the effect of treating his hallucinations and other psychotic symptons, but he now appears to be lethargic and lacking in drive, and communicates in a monotone. He is often restless and paces around much of the time with seeming little purpose.

This case study illustrates some of the common features of schizophrenia. Barry initially experienced strange thoughts and hallucinations. He later became increasingly withdrawn and lifeless.

NOTE: The case of Barry Horton will be referred to at different stages in these materials

WHAT IS SCHIZOPHRENIA?

Schizophrenia is a condition characterised by features such as hearing voices which are not there - but which are "real" to the person experiencing them - and having strange, tormenting and often paranoid ideas. (It is important to note, however, that not all people who hear voices have a diagnosis of schizophrenia, and not all people find their voices unpleasant at all times). For some, the symptoms of schizophrenia come in periods of illness lasting weeks or months, while for others there may be only occasional periods of relief. Schizophrenia is frequently disabling - for example, making it difficult to hold down a job - and often misunderstood.

Schizophrenia does not mean that the person has a split personality.

Activity

- *Ask friends, relatives and colleagues what they believe schizophrenia is, and write down their responses.*

- *How accurate were their responses?*

WHAT DOES THE FUTURE HOLD FOR THE INDIVIDUAL WITH A DIAGNOSIS OF DEPRESSION? (PROGNOSIS)

The short and long-term outlook for people with depression varies greatly. Although many experience a good short-term response to treatment, more than 70% later relapse, while approximately 20% will go on to develop a chronic condition. As many as 10-15% of people with moderate to severe depression commit suicide.

The likelihood of a poor long-term outcome is increased by low self-esteem, lack of social support or poor quality of support (for example, criticism by family members) and strongly held pessimistic ideas during the initial period of depression. In addition, people who were seen as excessively dependant before the onset of depression are more likely to have a poor outcome.

MODULE 1

MOOD (AFFECTIVE) DISORDERS
Manic-Depression

CASE STUDY: Dorothy

Dorothy is 50 years old, and has been divorced for 11 years. She lives with her mother who is in good health, and her student daughter. Dorothy is outgoing and "chatty" as a personality, and has many friends through her work as a receptionist for a large engineering company.

In recent weeks, Dorothy is described as having become unusually "moody", weeping at times, but rapidly recovering. In the past 2-3 days she has become excitable and has developed an enormous drive to redecorate and furnish the whole house. She ordered 300 metres of curtain material at an expensive store, and stayed up for three nights making curtains. When they were finished she declared them "not good enough" and ordered even more expensive fabric to replace them. To pay for it, she wrote cheques for enormous amounts, which the bank refused to honour. At work there have been episodes of unusual explosions of anger, and excitable, rapid and over-familiar conversations with business clients.

12 months on

In her first period of illness, Dorothy was admitted to hospital under the Mental Health Act, 1983, and treated with neuroleptic drugs. She recovered and returned to work, but has had two similar episodes since, which were highly disruptive of her family life. Following the second she lost her job. Her mother has become anxious and weary and is unable to sleep. She is being treated for raised blood pressure. She says she feels she is on a permanent "knife edge", and is terrified by the way Dorothy loses control when she is ill.

WHAT IS MANIC-DEPRESSION?

Manic-depression is a mental illness characterised by two extremes (or poles) of mood (you may therefore hear it referred to as **bipolar mood disorder**). These extremes are severe depression (sometimes psychotic in nature), and elation - mania. Mania, is a highly elated state of mind; a slightly milder form, hypomania, is more common. The individual suffering from manic-depression experiences episodes of depression and episodes of hypomania. Sometimes both depression and hypomania occur in the same period of illness. These episodes may last from a few days to several months.

Having already described the features of depression, we will focus in this section on the characteristics of hypomania.

WHAT MIGHT INDICATE THAT SOMEONE HAS HYPOMANIA?

The main features of hypomania are elation, rapid speech, tremendous energy, self-importance, a lack of inhibitions and seemingly untiring levels of energy. At first, when mania is mild, the individual seems to be in high spirits and his/her laughter can be infectious. As it progresses, however, the person's behaviour becomes exhausting. Some people who are hypomanic are so full of energy and ideas that they are irritable if challenged, and may become aggressive.

The key signs and symptoms may be categorised as follows:

- **Changes in mood, thoughts and feelings.**
- **Changes in general appearance and behaviour.**
- **Physical changes.**

Changes in Mood, Thoughts and Feelings

Thoughts increase in rate - mood is elated ("high") or irritable, and sometimes changeable, this may be evident from the person's speech, which is also fast. The individual's conversation may jump around from topic to topic as he/she tries to keep pace with an abundance of exciting - as the person sees it - ideas entering his/her mind **(flight of ideas)**. The person is self-important and over-confident of his or her abilities. Nothing is too big a task and yet the individual often does not have the patience to complete what has been started.

People with hypomania may be extravagant, spending money they do not have. Disinhibited behaviour may lead to problems at work, at home, or with the law. Driving can be affected by irritability, self-importance, distractibility.and poor judgement.

Example 1

Jane is currently hypomanic. She is full of energy and has decided to demonstrate her intelligence to the world by disproving Einstein's theories. At the end of the day Jane's husband returns home from work only to find the house filled with pieces of paper on which Jane had written jumbled mathematical symbols.

Example 2

Waseem was frequently in trouble with his bank-manager after he had experienced a period of hypomania. During his last episode, Waseem went out and purchased four new motor cars running up a bill of well over £40,000.

Delusions and hallucinations may also be experienced in severe cases, when they reflect the person's elated mood **(mood congruent)**. Like other thoughts, the delusions are often about grand plans, for example, to save the world. The person may believe he/she has supernatural powers, or has been chosen by God for some mission. The individual may believe he/she is a person of great importance, for example, a king **(grandiose delusions)**.

Example

Trevor believed that he was a superb author, and insisted that he was the great grand son of William Shakespeare. Despite the fact that most of his work was extremely muddled and almost impossible to understand, he sent it off to the publishers. He became extremely irate when he was immediately turned down.

The delusions may also be tormenting or threatening **(persecutory)**. Hallucinations are usually auditory, sometimes visual. The person may see visions or hear voices which reinforce his/her ideas of self-importance.

Example

Paul heard voices telling him that he was "The Chosen One" and choirs of angelic voices singing about him as God.

At the end of a period of hypomania, the person's mood either recovers or becomes depressed. Sometimes the depression is the result of realising the havoc that has been caused by the recent hypomania, which may have left him/her with serious debts or family problems or in trouble with the police.

Changes in General Appearance and Behaviour

The person's appearance and behaviour reflect his/her mood. The individual may be dressed in flamboyant or sexually provocative clothing. Make-up is bright and garish.

Physical Changes

The person is restless and his/her overactivity can cause physical exhaustion. Sleep is frequently disrupted in hypomania - because the person is so full of energy he/she does not seem to need it. If the individual does sleep, he/she will wake early, raring to get up and go and disturbing the household or neighbourhood.

Appetite is increased though sometimes the person is so overactive he/she has no time to stop and eat. Alcohol intake is also increased which may add to the problems. An increase in sexual desires and activity may also be seen, and the person may fail to take precautions against pregnancy or sexually transmitted diseases. Some embark on extramarital affairs.

THE PREVALENCE OF MANIC DEPRESSION?

Approximately 1% of the population will develop manic-depression at some point in their lives. It can begin at any time during adult life. Women are at a slightly higher risk.

WHAT CAUSES MANIC-DEPRESSION? (AETIOLOGY)

Inheritance (Genetic) Factors

There is strong evidence of a genetic basis to manic depression. Studies have shown that the immediate relatives (parents and siblings) of individuals with a diagnosis of manic-depression are around 24 times more likely to develop the condition than the average person.

Studies of identical twins, who, as mentioned previously, have the same genetic make-up, have shown that if one twin develops manic-depression, there is approximately a 68% chance that the other twin will also develop the condition. You may remember from the section on schizophrenia that if a condition was purely genetic and one identical twin suffered from it, the other twin would be at 100% risk of developing it also. Clearly, therefore, other factors must play a part.

Adoption studies have supported the importance of inheritance. Adopted children of parents with a diagnosis of manic-depression are at increased risk of developing the condition, in spite of the fact that they have been brought up in a different home environment from their natural parents. The genetic risk may be seen as another "vulnerability factor". Under certain adverse conditions, such as during stress or after childbirth, the vulnerable person may develop manic-depression.

Personality Factors

A particular type of personality is associated with an increased risk of developing manic-depression. This personality is described as "cyclothymic" and is characterised by mood swings that are less severe than those seen in manic-depression.

Physical Factors

Disturbance in the normal functioning of certain brain chemicals (**neurotransmitters**) underlies manic-depression. The chemicals are affected by antidepressant drugs which can cause hypomania in people who are depressed. Similarly, hormonal changes following childbirth, appear to act as a trigger of mania or depression in a syndrome called puerperal psychosis.

Life Events

As in depression, life events such as marriage or loss of a job, may bring about hypomania in those who were already vulnerable.

WHAT DOES THE FUTURE HOLD FOR THE INDIVIDUAL WITH A DIAGNOSIS OF MANIC-DEPRESSION?

There is a great deal of variation in the length of attacks of hypomania. For the majority the symptoms last several weeks or up to a few months. More rarely, recovery from the illness occurs within a few days. Once the person has experienced an episode of mania or depression, the frequency of his or her attacks may increase and they may get worse. On the other hand, some people recover after a single episode of mania or depression and never have another.

Activity

- Identify the genetic counselling services available in your area.
- What facilities do they provide for people who are concerned about the possibility of inheriting a mental health problem?

● ●

DILEMMA

Mr Simonedes is 55 years old and lives at home with his wife
and his eighteen year old son. He has had a number of
episodes of manic depressive illness, and takes regular
medication. On a routine visit, you notice that he is rather
more animated than usual, but not overtly ill. He tells you
that he has, on impulse, booked a flight to the USA to pursue
a "business hunch". His wife is very concerned, as she fears
a loss of judgement and knows his firm would not fund or
support this venture.

What might you do?

This may turn out to be a highly costly and damaging
expedition. It is likely that Mr Simonedes is becoming ill
again. On the other hand, he has the right to act on impulse.
This is clearly a complex dilemma involving the need to
balance individual rights with risks.

- Talk to Mrs. Simonedes in detail to identify
  sources of concern.

- Try to encourage Mr. Simonedes to see a doctor.

- Ask for a Mental Health Act assessment if the situation
  deteriorates, and Mr. Simonedes does not think he is ill.
  Discuss this with the relevant care manager and
  Approved Social Worker.

What other courses of action might you consider taking?

In the future it might be appropriate to plan with Mr. and Mrs.
Simonedes details of what action might be appropriate
should any similar situations occur in the future.

● ●

ANXIETY RELATED CONDITIONS

CASE STUDY: Marianne

Marianne had to give up work because of anxiety about meeting deadlines and the level of responsibility she was given. Over a period of several months, she was restless and had great difficulty sleeping. She was unable to concentrate and worried excessively about managing the social and practical demands of daily life.

Marianne has experienced feelings of panic when shopping in the supermarket. She becomes very tense and has to stand still because of sweating, shaking and a terror that she is about to die. She now avoids the supermarket because of these episodes. When she is outside her home she experiences a feeling of apprehension.

Marianne is suffering from a generalised anxiety disorder. She has also experienced panic attacks, such as the one in the supermarket and appears to be becoming phobic about leaving her home.

WHAT IS AN ANXIETY RELATED DISORDER?

We have all experienced periods of anxiety at some point in our lives: on our way to an interview; whilst waiting to hear important news; whilst taking a driving test and so on. In circumstances such as these it is seen as acceptable to "have butterflies", to feel tense and to be preoccupied with worries. These are all part of a normal "stress reaction".

A stress reaction is the body's response to difficult and testing situations and experiences. A series of body responses, both physical and psychological, occur during periods of stress, including:

PHYSICAL SYMPTOMS

- A "sickly" feeling (nausea), having "butterflies", or having diarrhoea
- The need to pass urine more frequently
- Dry mouth
- Sweating and hot flushes or "chilly" feelings
- Shaking, trembling or "legs like jelly"
- A feeling of one's heart thumping (palpitations) and an increase in heart rate (tachycardia)
- General bodily tension and muscular aches

PSYCHOLOGICAL SYMPTOMS

- Worry
- Apprehension
- Inability to think about anything else (inability to concentrate)
- Restlessness
- Fear

These symptoms are understandable in response to a "stressor", for example, being followed down a dark alley-way. They are also generally seen as acceptable if the individual remains able to function reasonably well "under the circumstances". They become an "anxiety disorder" when they increase in severity or are less understandable.

Under the rather general term of "anxiety disorders" fall a number of conditions, including:

- generalised anxiety disorder (GAD);
- panic disorder;
- phobias; and
- obsessive-compulsive disorder.

These anxiety symptoms are more severe forms of what most of us experience in everyday life, but additional symptoms also occur.

Anxiety symptoms also occur as part of depression, when the individual is restless and agitated. Depression may also be associated with panic attacks, phobias or obsessions.

WHAT MIGHT INDICATE THAT SOMEONE IS EXPERIENCING AN ANXIETY RELATED DISORDER?

A Generalised Anxiety Disorder

Some people find that they are anxious all or most of the time, but this does not mean that they suffer from generalised anxiety disorder. The symptoms experienced in a generalised anxiety disorder are much worse than "normal" anxiety and often occur in episodes. The individual with a generalised anxiety disorder will often have experienced some sort of upset prior to becoming anxious, but his/her anxiety persists long after the incident has passed.

Example
Mrs. Adams was the victim of a mugging six months ago. The mugger was caught and is currently in jail. Since the incident, however, Mrs. Adams continues to experience intense feelings of anxiety. Sometimes these feelings may last for several days.

Someone with a diagnoses of generalised anxiety disorder may experience the physical and mental symptoms of anxiety, as described before. During a period of anxiety, some individuals may also experience "panic attacks". When these are the main problem, the condition is referred to as "panic disorder" (see below)

Panic Disorder

Example
Mrs. Hurst was travelling on a bus to visit her grand children. Suddenly she developed intense feelings of fear. Her heart began to pound, her legs trembled and she felt hot and sweaty. She began to feel out of control and found that she was breathing very rapidly. She felt extremely anxious and had to get off the bus before she reached her stop.

This person has experienced a **panic attack** - a sudden episode of intense and uncontrollable fear. A client described this as "the feeling you might get if you were forced to walk a tightrope over the Niagara Falls".

The physical symptoms of anxiety are prominent in panic attacks. Frequently, individuals experience palpitations and a feeling that they are suffocating. Many over-breathe **(hyperventilate)** and this causes dizziness, pains, pins and needles and even greater feelings of breathlessness. Panicky thoughts make the symptoms worse. The person starts to think he/she is going to faint, have a heart attack, or die, and so becomes even more anxious.

Phobic Disorder

Individuals with a diagnosis of a phobic disorder become extremely anxious in a specific situation, for example, in the presence of spiders, or when travelling in a lift. The fear is so great that the person becomes anxious at the thought of the situation, and so avoids it.

Example
Jasmine, who suffers from a phobia of spiders (arachnophobia), is so terrified that she finds herself in a state of over-whelming anxiety when she sees anything to do with spiders. She was even anxious looking at the stalk on top of a tomato, as she believed that it looked like a spider.

The most disabling phobias are **social phobia** and, in particular, **agoraphobia**. In social phobia there is severe anxiety in social gatherings. The person feels that everyone is looking at him/her and is afraid of appearing foolish, blushing or being humiliated. The individual is afraid of being in public situations in which he/she has to eat or speak and so avoids these. In agoraphobia, anxiety occurs in open spaces such as an empty street, and crowded places, such as shops. Panic attacks often occur. Avoidance of shops, buses, or just being outside, can be so severe that the person can become as housebound as someone who is severely physically disabled.

Example

When Mrs. O'Neill developed agoraphobia she became very dependent on her daughter Charlotte. Initially she asked her to collect her benefit and to do her shopping. Recently however Mrs. O'Neill's agoraphobia has become more disabling. Charlotte now finds that she has to put her mothers rubbish into the dust-bin outside, as Mrs. O'Neill becomes extremely anxious when she goes into her back yard

Although these anxiety disorders have been described separately, it is often found that there is no clear dividing line between the conditions. For example, someone may have a diagnosis of generalised anxiety disorder, yet also experience phobias and panic attacks. Likewise, people with depression may also feel over-whelmed by feelings of generalised anxiety, or panic attacks and phobias. When depression and anxiety are experienced together, depression is usually treated as the underlying problem.

Obsessive-Compulsive Disorder (OCD)

Many of us will have had the experience of being unable to put a thought out of our minds. When such thoughts occur repeatedly and become distressing, they are known as **"obsessions"**.

It is also common to feel the need to 'check'. For example, having locked the door, you may feel a niggling doubt that you have not locked it and so you return to check. When this need to check something repeatedly is so severe that it begins to take over the individual's life, it is referred to as **"compulsive"**. In obsessive-compulsive disorder, the obsessive thought and compulsive behaviour are often linked.

Example

Mr. Rogers experiences an obsessive thought, that he is contaminated and desperately feels the need to wash his hands. This process continues throughout the day, sometimes compelling him to wash his hands several hundred times.

Four key features of obsessive compulsive disorder can be identified:

- **Intrusive thoughts** and **images** which are often of a disturbingly violent or sexual nature.

Example

Mrs. Graham experienced an image of herself picking up a knife and stabbing her family.

When such frightening thoughts and images are part of obsessive compulsive disorder, the individual does not usually act on them. If they are delusions (see page 10) they can be very dangerous.

- Constant brooding, obsessively turning worries over and over in one's mind **(ruminating)**

- **Compulsions**, for example, "checking" or repetitive hand washing.

- **Rituals** - the need to do things in a particular way. Some people have elaborate washing rituals that take them hours to complete. Others may have to count to a high number before crossing the road or entering a room.

Example

Before being able to do anything else in the day, Mr. Smith had to go through a lengthy routine of bathing and dressing. The other day, the telephone rang just as he was about to finish tying his shoe lace. He began to experience strong feelings of anxiety and had to put the 'phone down so that he could begin the process of bathing and dressing once again.

It is not difficult to see how restricted a person's life can become in obsessive compulsive disorder. Often the individual is tormented by obsessions and the compulsion to do things that appear strange to others.

THE PREVALENCE OF ANXIETY RELATED DISORDERS

Approximately 8% of the population have been identified as experiencing an anxiety disorder at any one time. Anxiety disorders are identified twice as often in women as in men.

MODULE 1

WHAT CAUSES ANXIETY RELATED DISORDERS TO DEVELOP?

Inheritance (Genetic) Factors

The search to discover whether anxiety related disorders are inherited has relied on studies of families and twins (see pages 11 and 12 for explanation).

- Generalised anxiety disorders have been found to be more common in individuals where there is a family history of the condition. Compared to a 3% chance of developing generalised anxiety disorders in the general population, the risk increases to around 15% in individuals where an immediate relative has been diagnosed with the condition. Identical twin studies have also shown a possible genetic link: the risk of one twin developing generalised anxiety disorders if the other has been diagnosed is around 41%.

- Panic disorder, also, appears to have an inherited component. In the general population, approximately 6% develop panic disorder, compared to approximately 12% of those whose immediate relatives are diagnosed with the condition. Identical twin studies have shown that if one twin develops a panic disorder, the risk for the other twin is around 35-40 %.

- Phobia - The first degree relatives of individuals who suffer from phobias are more likely to develop a phobia than the rest of the general population. Where a parent or sibling suffers with social phobia, the immediate relatives have been found to have at least a threefold increase in risk. Similarly, agoraphobia is believed to have a strong genetic origin. Although there does appear to be an increased chance of developing phobias in the immediate relatives of those with simple phobias, the evidence is not as clear as in agoraphobia and social phobia.

- Obsessive-compulsive disorder - Research into the genetics of obsessive compulsive disorders is at an early stage. To date, however, there appears to be some indication that obsessive compulsive disorder is also partly inherited. One study found that if a parent or sibling was diagnosed as having obsessive compulsive disorder, the risk of the immediate relatives developing

the condition was high: 23% of immediate family members displaying characteristic symptoms. Other studies have found that an immediate relative of a person diagnosed with obsessive compulsive disorder was twice as likely as the rest of the general population to develop any anxiety related disorder, (not necessarily obsessive compulsive disorder).

Physical Causes

The fact that panic attacks often occur "out of the blue", has been taken as evidence that they may have a biological cause. It is believed that in some individuals who suffer from panic disorder and other anxiety conditions, the biological mechanisms for arousal are unstable. A lack of one neurotransmitter - **serotonin**, has been suggested as a possible cause in the development of anxiety related conditions.

Physical ill-health may at times be seen to trigger the onset of anxiety, perhaps because illnesses are threatening life events. Several studies have identified the onset of anxiety disorders following the development of a physical condition or surgery .

Personality

People with certain types of personality appear to be at greater risk of developing anxiety related disorders. In particular, those who are more than usually anxious are at increased risk.

Psychological Theories

Several complex theories have been put forward to explain why individuals develop anxiety related disorders. The main ones are outlined below. For further reading, an introductory psychology textbook should be consulted.

Learned Behaviour

According to the learning theories, the individual learns (or is conditioned) to behave in certain ways. The following example best illustrates " conditioning"

Example

The office Beth was in was set on fire. She found the experience harrowing although she was not physically injured. At the time of the emergency she heard fire alarms ringing and the sirens of fire engines. Several months later she became concerned as she found herself experiencing severe symptoms of anxiety whenever the fire alarm sounded for a rehearsal at work. Indeed whilst shopping recently she heard a fire engine pass with its sirens screaming out. She became so anxious that she began hyperventilating and eventually fainted. She has now altered her route home from work so that she does not drive anywhere near to the fire station.

This person has learned to associate sirens and bells with the intense feelings of fear and anxiety experienced during the fire. By avoiding the situation, she is seen to be reinforcing her fears - making them worse by not facing them.

Cognitive Theory

According to cognitive theory, the individual experiences a pattern of anxious thoughts when in certain situations that make the person uneasy. These thoughts are more fearful, and a vicious circle develops in which the more anxious the person feels, the more thoughts of disaster occur to him, and vice versa.

Psycho-analytic

Sigmund Freud (a psychoanalyst and a doctor), based his theory on his experience of studying women with "hysteria" (an apparent physical illness which has a psychological cause). He suggested that the anxiety these women suffered came from their struggle to suppress strong feelings, for example, hatred or sexual desire that they could not accept. Although his numerous theories played an important part in the history of psychiatry, they are less influential in clinical practice today.

Attachment

This theory suggests that anxiety results from either the lack of an attachment during early childhood, or from a child's difficulties in developing a close and trusting relationship with its main carer. A child is said to become insecure

without a parent to depend upon. In later life, the individual is vulnerable to anxiety at times of loss or separation because these revive childhood insecurities.

Life-Events

Stressful life events may provoke an episode of generalised anxiety disorder, particularly in someone who is already vulnerable, for example, someone with an anxious personality. If a person faces stressful social circumstances after the development of generalised anxiety disorder these may delay recovery.

WHAT DOES THE FUTURE HOLD FOR THE INDIVIDUAL WITH A DIAGNOSIS OF AN ANXIETY RELATED DISORDER?

Generalised Anxiety Disorder

Anxiety disorders that are directly related to particular stresses are likely to recover quickly. About 50% of people recover within a month. Some people, however, especially those who are referred to mental health services, go on to develop depression. In others, the recovery is slow, although this depends on such factors as social circumstances and personality.

Panic Disorder

The long-term outlook for a person diagnosed with this condition varies widely. Some people find that their symptoms disappear after only a few weeks. Others find that they have a long term problem and experience periods where their panic attacks are frequent and disabling.

Phobic Disorder

The recovery from phobic disorder depends to a large extent on the type of phobia experienced. Simple phobias (for example, fear of spiders) are usually treatable. Social phobias tend to begin in early adult life and often get better. Agoraphobia, also develops in young adults about this time. The outlook for people who develop agoraphobia is worse - symptoms may recur and or become long-term **(chronic)**. About 60% of phobic patients seeing psychiatrists have agoraphobia - not because it is the most common, but because it is the most disabling and difficult to treat.

Obsessive-Compulsive Disorder

If the individual has no underlying obsessive personality disorder the outlook is better (see page 34 for an explanation of this personality disorder). It is generally accepted that around two-thirds of people who suffer from obsessive compulsive disorder will recover within a year. For the remainder there will be periods without symptoms **(remission)** and then times during which the intrusive thoughts and urges return **(relapse)**.

People diagnosed with anxiety related disorders are found to have high death rates because of suicide and heart disease (possibly due to the effects of smoking).

DEMENTIA

CASE STUDY: Mr Lee

Mr. Lee is 79 years of age and lives at home with his wife. He retired from his career as a senior executive within a retail business at the age of 65 and has since enjoyed a healthy retirement.

Over the last year or so, however, Mr. Lees' golfing friends have noticed that "his memory appears to be failing him". Previously Mr. Lee had never failed to miss an arranged game, but over the past few months he has missed several due to his forgetfulness. At home his wife feels that Mr. Lee is becoming increasingly confused. Sometimes he appears to forget where he is, at other times he cannot remember the names of members of his family and his friends.

More recently, Mr. Lee appears to be showing little interest in his appearance. His wife now has to remind him to take a bath and comb his hair. Mrs. Lee regards this as a sign that "something just isn't right. He's always looked so well turned-out. I've never seen him neglect himself like this before".

Last week Mrs. Lee discussed the situation with her sons. They too felt that there had been a gradual change in Mr. Lee's behaviour and appearance over the past two years and suggested that Mrs. Lee should ask the GP to visit.

The above case demonstrates some of the symptoms commonly experienced in the early stages of dementia.

WHAT IS DEMENTIA?

Dementia is a syndrome, the most characteristic signs and symptoms of which include memory loss and personality changes. The most common forms of dementia are Alzheimer's disease and multi-infarct dementia. Although we all experience changes in our mental abilities, in dementia these changes become so severe that they affect an individual's ability to function in normal daily life.

At times you may hear the terms "pre-senile dementia" and "senile dementia". These are not diagnoses, but simply refer to the age at which the individual develops the condition. If the person begins to suffer from the condition before the age of sixty-five this is described as "pre-senile dementia" after this age it is referred to as "senile dementia".

WHAT MIGHT INDICATE THAT AN INDIVIDUAL IS SUFFERING FROM DEMENTIA?

The following signs and symptoms are characteristic of dementia:

- **Memory problems and changes in intelligence**
- **Personality and behaviour changes**
- **Physical changes**
- **Mood disorders**
- **Hallucinations and delusions**

Memory Problems and Changes in Intelligence

The loss of memory often develops gradually at first and may go unnoticed for a period, the changes being put down to "old age".

Example
Mrs. Bates went on a Christmas shopping trip to York with the other members of a Nottingham Bridge group. Later that night when she returned, she telephoned her daughter. In the midst of the conversation, Mrs. Bates became particularly irritated by the fact that she was completely unable to recall the name of the city she had just visited.

As the condition progresses, however, clear difficulties in memory may be seen, especially for events which have happened recently **(short-term memory loss)**. The person struggles to come up with words, becomes confused and is unable to deal with his or her usual daily activities. He/she often becomes disorientated, and may be found wandering around, lost in surroundings which were previously familiar.

Intelligence, initiative and the ability to reason are all progressively affected. Thoughts slow down and the individual may find it difficult to understand what is happening.

Personality and Behaviour Changes

The individual's character and behaviour change dramatically as the decline in mental ability continues. The person gradually appears to lose touch with his/her social surroundings, at times behaving in ways considered by others to be inappropriate or out of character, or failing to observe normal social rules and "manners". He or she may experience episodes of anger and aggression as a result of minor frustrations **(catastrophic reaction)**, although often there is no clear reason why the outburst should suddenly occur (see "mood disorders" below).

Such changes in behaviour and attitude to life are particularly distressing for friends and relatives as they watch someone they know change beyond recognition.

"Sometimes it is as if the true self dies long before the body's death, and in the intervening years a smudged caricature disintegrates noisily and without dignity into chaos."[5]

Physical Changes

The changes which occur throughout the brain may lead to problems with speech and movement. Some people find difficulty in carrying out movements even though they know what they want to do **(dyspraxia)**. People with multi-infarct dementia have poor blood supply to the brain, and this can cause paralysis or loss of balance.

In the later stages of dementia, incontinence of urine and faeces may also occur. This is particularly stressful for family carers.

Mood Disorders

In the early stages of dementia, the person has some insight into what is happening and often understands what degrading changes may be in store for them. During this period, depression, anxiety and frustration are common. Suicide is sometimes considered. As the condition progresses, and the person becomes less aware of circumstances and surroundings, his/her mood often becomes "flat" and unemotional. At times, however the person may experience sudden outbursts of laughter or anger, which appear to arise "out of the blue".

Delusions and Hallucinations

These do not always occur, but if they do, they take the form of "voices" **(auditory hallucinations)** and beliefs that others are tormenting them **(persecutory delusions)**. To refresh your memory on delusions and hallucinations, please turn to pages 9 to 10.

Activity

- **Identify the problems you might anticipate for the close relatives of people suffering from dementia?**

- **In your area what facilities are available for these carers?**

THE PREVALENCE OF DEMENTIA

Dementia is a growing problem because of the increase in average life expectancy. It is currently found to affect around 5-10% of people over 65 years old, increasing to around 25-30 % of those over 80 years old. Alzheimer's disease (named after Alois Alzheimer who first identified the condition), is the commonest form of dementia, affecting around 60% of sufferers. Multi-infarct dementia affects between 20-30%.

Other, much rarer forms of dementia are those which result from conditions which directly affect the brain. These include vitamin deficiency, hypothyroidism, brain tumours, brain damage (for example, as a result of boxing injuries) and infection (for example Creutzfeld-Jacob disease).

WHAT CAUSES DEMENTIA TO DEVELOP?

Alzheimer's Disease

People with this type of dementia have a characteristic form of damage to their brain tissue. A substantial number of nerve cells break down or **degenerate** and the damaged nerve cells are described as **tangles** or **plaques** depending on their appearance under the microscope. In normal ageing, plaques and tangles are found in far smaller amounts. Alzheimer's disease is not, therefore, just an extreme form of ageing.

There are several theories why these changes may occur:

Inheritance Factors

The risk of developing Alzheimer's disease is increased if there is a strong family history of the condition. Studies on identical twins, sharing the same biological make-up, have shown that if one twin develops the condition, the chance of the other twin also doing so is around 50% (to refresh your memory on the significance of twin studies, refer back to pages 11 and 12).

In studies of high risk families, a specific genetic abnormality has been identified as linked to Alzheimer's. This fact is important as it may begin to tell scientists more about the biological mechanisms of the disease.

Effect of Aluminium

Aluminium is seen in the plaques and tangles found in brain tissue in Alzheimer's disease. It has, therefore, been suggested that an excess of aluminium in the body may lead to an increased risk of developing the condition. The results of studies exploring this possibility have proved inconclusive.

Down's Syndrome

Individuals born with Down's Syndrome, a condition caused by a genetic abnormality, have been found to develop premature aging of the brain, similar to that seen in Alzheimer's disease.

Multi-Infarct Dementia (MID)

The brain tissue of people who suffer from MID shows patchy damage. This is caused by minute blockages in the blood supply to nerve cells which result in their death. The area of damage is called an **infarct**, and in MID numerous tiny infarcts occur. Strokes occur in the same way as this, only the damage is more sudden and affects a large area, for example, the part of the brain controlling movement.

Blood vessels in the brain become blocked more easily if they are affected by arteriosclerosis. In this condition the walls of blood vessels become thick, hard and fatty. This obstructs the circulation in many parts of the body, but is particularly dangerous in the heart and brain. Several factors are believed to increase the risk of developing arteriosclerosis and therefore make MID more likely. These include: high blood pressure; diabetes; smoking; a poor diet; lack of exercise; age; male sex and genetic influences (for example, a familial tendency to high blood cholesterol levels).

WHAT DOES THE FUTURE HOLD FOR THE INDIVIDUAL WITH A DIAGNOSIS OF DEMENTIA?

Dementia affects people in different ways. Alzheimer's disease appears to start more slowly than multi-infarct dementia. The progress of MID is sometimes described as "stepwise", which refers to the way in which each new episode of damage (each infarct) adds to the deterioration in the person's condition.

Regardless of which type of dementia is experienced, the outlook is generally poor. Death is likely within two to five years. In the case of MID the cause of death may be heart disease, because both are caused by poor circulation

DILEMMA

Mr. Taylor is a 72 year old retired post office clerk. His wife died 8 years ago and he has lived alone ever since. He has no relatives locally. You are a support worker and have been working with Mr. Taylor over the past year, since he developed dementia. Home care workers help him with cleaning and shopping, and you visit fortnightly to monitor his progress and offer support. You feel that you have built up a strong and trusting relationship with him. Over the past few months his memory appears to have been getting worse and he is accusing home care workers of stealing from him. Today, for the first time, he has accused you.

What might you do?

- Clearly the first point to make is that any accusation should be taken seriously and investigated. All staff need to accept the necessity for this.

- In situations such as these, it is also important to ensure that the care manager is kept fully informed and that guidelines, such as signing for financial transactions, are followed. It might be worth requesting that the finances within the house are kept to a minimum, providing Mr. Taylor gives permission. In some situations it may be necessary to visit the client in pairs.

- Concerns about Mr. Taylor's failing memory should be discussed with the care manager. If he is forgetting where he has put his money he might be at risk personally. He could, for example, forget to turn the gas off or begin wandering out of the house at night - a case review should therefore be arranged.

- Additional services may be helpful, for example, does Mr. Taylor attend any day care services? Circumstances such as these are distressing for all the staff involved and support should be offered by the care manager. It may also be helpful for the support staff to get together and openly discuss their feelings. It is important for a positive and supportive view to be maintained towards Mr. Taylor (his use of services will progressively increase).

Consider what other courses of action you might have considered taking?

PERSONALITY DISORDERS

CASE STUDY: Carly

Carly is 26 years old and is a lone parent of four children aged 8 years, 7 years, 3 years and 21 months.

Carly spent much of her early life in care, following physical and suspected sexual abuse by her step-father. Carly lived in a number of different children's homes and foster homes, and the records reveal a pattern of increasingly problematic behaviour.

In her early teens, Carly began running away and missing school. She was placed on probation for setting fire to a school when she was 15 years old. Carly became pregnant at 17 years of age, and married her boyfriend (who also had a care history). They had two children, but then parted following the husband's imprisonment following a robbery.

Carly has since had several relationships with men, and is unsure who the father of her fourth child is.

Carly continues to be the concern of many agencies. Her children are all on the Child Protection Register, due to incidents when Carly had left them alone overnight. The two youngest have had hospital admissions following domestic accidents. Carly denies any difficulties with the children and says that neighbours and friends are to blame for "letting her down".

Carly has harmed herself on several occasions in moments of crisis, and has been admitted twice to a psychiatric unit on a section of the Mental Health Act, 1983. However, these incidents become meaningless to her once the crisis is over.

Carly is subject to a probation order for fraud and illegal reconnection of a meter.

Carly has poor relationships with family and friends, and her relationships with professionals are fraught. She perceives people as being "for or against her", and cannot tolerate any challenge. She refuses to talk to social workers since the children were put on the Child Protection Register. She makes excessive demands on other professionals for support.

Because of escalating concerns about the welfare and development of the four children, it is likely that the children will be removed into the care of the local authority under an order of the Children Act, 1989. Her housing tenure is also in jeopardy because of rent debt, and complaints from neighbours about the behaviour of visitors to the home.

Carly is described as having a "personality disorder".

WHAT ARE PERSONALITY DISORDERS?

The word "personality" refers to all of those qualities which make an individual unique, including the way a person thinks, feels and behaves. Features of personality are known as "traits" and groups of traits that often go together form a personality type. We often describe ourselves or others in terms of these traits.

Example

"Natalie is always so self-centred and vain, but I do wish I had her confidence".

Some types of personality cause regular problems either to the person concerned or to others and may be diagnosed as a Personality Disorder (PD), for example, a person too anxious to sustain a relationship or too impulsive to hold down a job without walking out. Some believe that this category of mental health problems has been reserved for people whose diagnosis is uncertain or who are difficult to engage in treatment. It is notoriously difficult to define the boundary between 'personality disorder' and the 'normal' range of personality.

In a person with personality disorder such traits as, for example, paranoia (or unusual suspiciousness) are part of the enduring personality structure and therefore less likely to be affected by treatment. In severe mental illness, paranoia may take the form of a delusion, which is not part of the individual's normal experience and may respond to treatment.

WHAT MIGHT INDICATE THAT SOMEONE HAS A PARTICULAR TYPE OF PERSONALITY DISORDER?

Personality disorders commonly encountered by health and social services staff are "antisocial" and "borderline" PD. You may therefore hear these terms referred to more frequently than the other personality disorders described below. The purpose of the following descriptions is to help the learner recognise personality disorders and provide appropriate services for users with this diagnosis. Care should be taken that the descriptions provided do not become negative value judgements and labels.

- **Antisocial** (originally referred to as "psychopathic") - impulsive, callous, self-centred and shameless. Individuals with an anti-social PD are often disloyal in friendships, showing little sensitivity for the feelings of others. Difficulties in forming or maintaining personal relationships occur. Such individuals feel no guilt, even after cruel and hurtful acts towards others. The person's lack of restraint and inability to learn by mistakes often result in criminal offences.

- **Borderline** - A number of disordered personality traits are seen in individuals with this diagnosis. Their moods often appear unstable, and there are outbursts of anger, periods of depression and episodes of "normality". The intensity of mood experienced is extreme. They are often impulsive, which frequently results in antisocial behaviour such as lying, stealing, gambling and drug and alcohol abuse. People with borderline PD often inflict direct harm on themselves by self-cutting or overdose. They may also be excessively dependent, and afraid of loss or abandonment.

The key characteristics of some of the other personality disorders are described below.

- **Schizoid** A person who presents as shy, introverted, and emotionally cold. These individuals prefer their own company, withdrawing from social situations and often failing to develop friendships or relationships. They often lack a sense of humour and appear to be cut off from the world around them.

- **Paranoid** An individual who presents as suspicious, unable to trust and thin-skinned. The person with a paranoid personality is suspicious that others are out to humiliate or hurt him/her. The person also has strong feelings of self-importance and may blame any failure experienced on those he or she considers "untrustworthy".

- **Histrionic** A person who presents as self-centred, attention-seeking and intense. People displaying this personality disorder behave as if "all the world's a stage". They draw attention to themselves by over-dramatising their lives and this often results in stormy relationships. They may use displays of emotion to manipulate others, for example, by threatening suicide.

- **Obsessive-compulsive** The individual who presents as painstaking, inflexible, constantly "checking"'. Such people are driven by a need to feel secure and in control, and display a tiresome preoccupation with routine. Their strong desire to stick to rules results in intolerance of the seemingly "lax" behaviour of others. As a result, they are often viewed as judgemental and rigid.

- **Avoidant** The person who presents as anxious, excessively self-conscious and edgy. Such individuals are constantly afraid of rejection and concerned with what other people might think about them. This uneasiness affects their lives to such an extent that they avoid placing themselves in situations or relationships where they may be criticised or challenged. This makes it difficult to enter a relationship or seek a new job and so on.

- **Dependent** The individual who presents as lacking in self-confidence, passive and indecisive. These individuals are often considered weak and unassertive, only too pleased to fall in line with the wishes of others rather than "standing on their own two feet." Their reluctance to take charge of their own lives ultimately leaves them unable to cope independently.

- **Narcissistic** The person who presents as self-absorbed and insensitive to the feelings of others. Such people are filled with ideas of self-importance and pride. Their inflated self-interest and constant need for praise leaves them unable to recognise the needs of others. Difficulties in relationships may therefore arise.

- **Impulsive** The individual who presents as instinctive, rash and likely to "blow a fuse" . Individuals with an impulsive PD fail to consider the consequences of their actions beforehand. Their anger often appears to be out of control as they rise to situations without any fore-thought. They may also be considered to be argumentative and moody. They run into difficulties in employment and relationships, or with the law, which they often regret later.

HOW COMMON ARE PERSONALITY DISORDERS?

It has been suggested that as many as 10% of the population may have a personality disorder (although only a minority of these will come to the attention of mental health services). Anti-social personality disorder is believed to affect 2-3% of the population, while approximately 1% of the population are believed to have a borderline personality disorder. Anti-social and obsessive PDs are more common in men, while borderline and depressive PDs are more common in women.

WHAT CAUSES THE DEVELOPMENT OF A PERSONALITY DISORDER?

What leads to the development of a personality disorder is not yet fully understood. Most of the research to date has focussed on antisocial personality disorder because of the destructive impact such individuals may have on society. Some of the major factors believed to be associated with a PD are outlined below.

Inheritance (Genetic) and Biological Factors

Inheritance plays a part in the development of some personality disorders. In particular, the close family of individuals with schizoid, paranoid, obsessive-compulsive and antisocial personality disorders appear to be at greater risk of developing a personality disorder.

The biological basis of personality traits is not well understood but there is much interest in the brain neurotransmitter **serotonin** which may be required for impulse control. Disorders of the way serotonin works may therefore, lie behind impulsive behaviour.

Psychological and Social Factors

There is evidence that adverse childhood experiences can influence the development of personality. The exact mechanisms by which this happens are not known, but poor self-esteem in children who are mistreated, and observational learning in children who witness constant aggression are likely to be important.

WHAT DOES THE FUTURE HOLD FOR SOMEONE WITH A DIAGNOSIS OF A PERSONALITY DISORDER?

Personality is by definition an enduring characteristic and therefore, dramatic changes are unlikely. It appears however, that with increasing age, personality disorders do tend to become less severe. Several reasons for these changes have been suggested:

- there may be changes of neurotransmitters with increasing age;

- alternative coping styles may be learned with greater experience of life;

- stressful home situations may change, for example, children may grow up and leave the home .

Rates of death by accidents and by suicide appear to be increased in individuals with personality disorders. The increase in accidental death may be because such individuals are prepared to take risks.

Personality disorder is one of the most common diagnoses found in individuals who have committed suicide. The risk of death by suicide is particularly high for those with borderline PD, in whom it has been found to be around 15%.

Activity

How responsive do you think your agency is in meeting the needs of people with personality disorders?

MODULE 1

References

1 World Health Organization (1992) *The ICD-10 Classification of Mental and Behavioural Disorders: Clinical Descriptions and Diagnostic Guidelines.* Geneva: WHO.

2 Bayley R. (1993) Hear our Voices. *Nursing Times.* Vol 89, 32-33.

3 Schiller L. (1992) Waking from the Nightmare of Schizophrenia. *Journal of Psychological Nursing and Mental Health Services.* Vol. 30 No. 5 Pg. 48.

4 Brown G. W. And Harris T. O. (1978) *Social Origins of Depression.* London: Tavistock.

5 Pitt B. (1982) *Psychogeriatrics. An Introduction to the Psychiatry of Old Age.* London: Churchill Livingstone.

Further Reading

Brown G.W. & Harris T.O.(Eds.) (1989) *Life Events and Illness.* London: Unwin Hyman Ltd.

Gelder MG., Gath D., Mayou R., & Cowen P., (1996) *The Textbook of Psychiatry.* Oxford: Oxford University Press.

Goldberg D., Benjamin S. & Creed F. (1994) (2nd ed) *Psychiatry in Medical Practice.* London and New York: Routledge.

Goldberg D., & Huxley P. (1980) *Mental Illness in the Community. The Pathway to Psychiatric Care.* London: Tavistock.

Newton J. (1988) *Preventing Mental Illness.* London: Routledge.

Paykel E.S. & Priest R.G. (1992) Recognition and Management of Depression in General Practice: Consensus Statement. *British Medical Journal,* 305: 1198-202.

Vaughn C. & Leff J. (1976) The Influence of Family and Social Factors on the Course of Psychiatric Illness. *British Journal of Psychiatry* 129 125-137.

Warner R. (1994) *Recovery from Schizophrenia.* London: Routledge.

• •

This module - "Recognition of Mental Health Problems" - is one of 7 modules in "Learning Materials on Mental Health - An Introduction". The other modules include:

Module 2 - "Intervention and Management"
Module 3 - "Legislation and Guidance"
Module 4 - "Special Client Groups"
Module 5 - "Special Issues"
Module 6 - "Users, Carers and Children of Parents with Mental Health Problems"
Module 7 - "Sample Training Exercises"

A sister set of materials is also available for professionals involved in assessing risk - "Learning Materials on Mental Health Risk Assessment"

module 2

INTERVENTION AND MANAGEMENT

....

AIMS & OBJECTIVES

After you have worked through this module you should be better able to:

- Describe the pathways of referral to the mental health services.

- Identify the places where individuals with mental health problems may attend for treatment/support.

- Describe the range of drug treatments available and their effects.

- Describe the various psychological interventions available.

SYSTEMS THROUGH WHICH INTERVENTIONS ARE DELIVERED

MODULE 2

THE CARE PROGRAMME APPROACH (CPA) AND CARE MANAGEMENT

These are now the central systems for organizing social and specialist health care services for people experiencing mental health problems. People who have been referred to specialist mental health services should receive support organised under the CPA. The CPA involves:

- **The assessment of the client's social and health care needs**
- **The drawing up of a package of care**
- **The identification of a key worker**
- **Regular monitoring and review of the client's needs**

The level of support and intervention required is assessed in accordance with the client's needs - **a needs assessment**. Needs may be defined as problems that the client is experiencing which can potentially be met by health and social interventions. Needs might exist in a number of areas:

- mental health
- physical health
- culture and spirituality
- day-time occupation
- housing
- money
- legal concerns
- day to day coping
- carers' difficulties.

Some people may be assessed as needing the full support of several members of the multi-disciplinary team, whilst others may only need a limited amount of support. Following an assessment of need a **package of care** and **care plan** are developed with the client, the carers (where relevant) and the members of the multidisciplinary team.

Under the CPA a **key worker** is nominated. Key workers could include social workers and community psychiatric nurses. The key worker is the member of the team who is directly responsible for ensuring that the interventions outlined in the client's care plan are working successfully. Key workers are in a position to develop close and trusting relationships with clients and may therefore provide essential feedback to the team on the appropriateness or success of the planned care. In situations where aspects of the package of care are inappropriate for the client, it is the key worker's responsibility to report such problems to the rest of the team.

Once a package of care has been developed and is in use, it is essential to hold regular reviews with the client and other members of the team in order to re-assess needs and to adapt the package of care accordingly.

The focus of the CPA is the client and his/her involvement in decision making is crucial to the success of the planning and delivery of care.

Within local authority Social Services Departments, care to vulnerable adults is organised through the system of **care management**. For adults with mental health problems this system should be integrated with the CPA, to provide a system within which both health and social care needs can be addressed.

Care management includes a number of tasks:

- **publishing information**
- **assessing needs**
- **care planning**
- **monitoring and review**
- **close involvement with users and carers**

Users/carers need to know what the result of the assessment is and details of services to be provided. The care plan should indicate what services are to be delivered.

The care manager is responsible for the assessment of needs and the organisation of care packages within the available resources. Local authorities have been encouraged to separate purchaser and provider functions within social services departments, with care management generally located on the purchaser side. The care manager's main task is to coordinate the services needed within a budget. There is encouragement to purchase services in the independent and voluntary sectors.

However, in mental health care, the services may be delivered more flexibly. Care managers are often ASWs or other social workers with a range of therapeutic skills. It may be appropriate for them to offer a direct and continuing service to individual clients, as well as acting in the roles of assessor and purchaser.

Patterns of care management vary between authorities. Sometimes the designated "care manager" will be responsible for assessment and the organisation of care, but will not offer ongoing involvement. At other times, "care managers" will both organise the services and maintain a supportive relationship with the service user and carers.

(See Module 3, *NHS and Community Care Act*, 1990).

CASE EXAMPLE OF THE CARE PROGRAMME APPROACH AT WORK - Barry Horton's case - continued from page 8.

When Barry Horton was last admitted to hospital he was experiencing disturbing hallucinations and had just begun taking antipsychotic medication. At the time of his admission, Barry was assessed by the multi-disciplinary team under the Care Programme Approach. Barry's needs and those of his parents' were assessed at this stage and a "package of care" was developed with Barry's involvement. A key worker, Clive, who was a community psychiatric nurse (CPN), was already working with Barry in the community. Clive worked closely with Barry and was responsible for ensuring the coordination of services within the "package of care". Key resources were accessed via care management arrangements.

During the time Barry was in hospital he started to appear increasingly lethargic and lacking in drive. His speech appeared monotonous. Barry's parents were pleased to hear that Barry's hallucinations were not troubling him as much as they had, but they were concerned to see him restlessly pacing around with seemingly little purpose. Barry had also asked Clive whether he could be discharged. A care programme review meeting was held to coordinate discharge planning and the ongoing multi-disciplinary assessment of Barry's needs and those of his parents. Barry's level of "risk" was also assessed in terms of both risk to himself and to others.

Assessed Needs Included:

Mental Health

- Barry is currently experiencing negative symptoms of schizophrenia. He feels unmotivated but somewhat agitated. He also feels he has lost confidence in himself.

- Barry has previously experienced disturbing hallucinations - these appear to have been suppressed following treatment with antipsychotic medication - which is currently being reduced onto a maintenance dose.

- Following a risk assessment by the psychiatrist, Barry is thought to be at low risk of harming others or himself - but he is thought to be at risk of self neglect.

Physical Health and Daily Living Activities

- Barry is lethargic and withdrawn at present - on the ward he has to be encouraged to eat, drink and attend to his hygiene needs.

- At night Barry finds that he is not sleeping well.

Social Needs

- Due to his current symptoms, Barry is unmotivated and does not wish to socialise with others on the ward. He feels he would be happier at home "where there is peace and quiet" and he doesn't have to see anyone if he doesn't want to.

- On discharge Barry is to return to his parents home.

Religious Needs

- Barry is a Catholic and used to attend his church regularly. Recently he has not felt able to go to church and he feels guilty about this.

Educational and Occupational Needs

- Prior to his present episode, Barry had been developing his long-standing interest in art and information technology, by accessing college based adult learning courses. These interests have waned recently due to increasing mental health difficulties.

Carers' Needs

- Barry's parents feel frustrated by the current situation. Although they have been given a full explanation as to why Barry is currently experiencing the negative symptoms, they do not appear reassured and are concerned about the effects of the antipsychotic medication.

- Barry's father works several miles from home and is currently concerned about threatened redundancies at work. He feels he cannot offer the support he would like to offer and is concerned about his wife and whether "she will cope".

- Barry's mother does not drive and she therefore wants to be certain that arrangements will be made for Barry to attend services on discharge.

It is decided that Barry is to be discharged. He will return to his parents home with an agreed package of care. This will combine both direct services and services purchased through care management. Clive, as key worker, will coordinate the delivery of these services and monitor their usefulness.

Package of Care:

Social Interventions

- Clive is to make arrangements for Barry to attend the local day hospital 3 days a week.

- At the day hospital assessment will continue, focusing upon Barry's current level of concentration and motivation.

- The Social Services Department are to arrange for a support worker to be identified through care management. Intervention will be:
  - *focused*
  - *flexible*
  - *low key and regular*
  - *coordinated and reviewed*

- The support worker will work with Barry to:
  - *develop a relationship*
  - *facilitate linkage with the community*
  - *enable independent living skills*
  - *enhance social skills*
  - *promote and monitor personal hygiene*
  - *facilitate re-engagement with adult learning courses*
  - *directly support Barry, providing reassurance and promoting confidence*

- Adult education learning course fees and associated costs are to be met from care management.

- Barry has agreed that he would like to contact his local priest again and his worker has offered to make the arrangements for this.

Physical Interventions

- Barry's mother will work with the support worker to minimise any problems in relation to Barry's hygiene and other daily living needs - the aim being to promote his independent living skills.

- Clive is to arrange for transport to the hospital to ensure Barry can attend his psychiatric out-patient appointments for review of his medication and mental health.

- Barry does not wish to receive additional medication to help him sleep - he feels that when he returns home the problem may well disappear. He agrees that this should be reviewed if he continues to experience problems sleeping.

Psychological Intervention

- Barry's psychological needs will be further assessed at the day hospital and relevant treatment will be planned if it is felt to be appropriate.

Carer's Intervention

- Clive and the support worker will jointly assess both Barry's parents' needs and the overall situation.

- Clive is to visit Barry's parents during the following week to offer reassurance and spend time answering any additional queries they may have following Barry's discharge. In addition, Clive will provide Barry's parents with information relating to their son's diagnosis, prognosis and plan of care.

Unmet Needs

- Unfortunately in Barry's local area there are no formal services available at the weekend, therefore, Barry's social needs may not be met. It is, however, hoped that Barry's re-introduction to the church may help with this problem, by providing informal support at weekends.

6 Month Review

Barry's mental health has been stable and he is to be discharged from the day hospital. Meaningful contact has developed with the support worker and this has achieved re-engagement with adult education courses and a gradual switch to a community based day service facility. This provides structure to his time and continues to give his mother some respite.

The local priest has been helpful and supportive. Barry is regularly attending Sunday services, and is also using a church drop-in for unemployed young people which offers him some social outlets, sports and activities.

Barry's medication is working well. His symptoms are well controlled, and he is experiencing few side effects. The psychiatrist will keep this under review at Barry's regular out-patient appointment, but no changes are needed at this time.

The above case example demonstrates how the key worker, in this case Clive, a CPN, is involved in both supporting the client and carers directly and in organising services to meet Barry's and his parents' needs. The services provided within the package of care include social, psychological and physical interventions which are provided by members of a multi-disciplinary mental health care team. Some services (for example, the support worker and the local day centre) are provided via social services care management arrangements.

THE SPECTRUM OF MENTAL HEALTH SERVICES

INTRODUCTION

For many people experiencing mental health problems, their GP will be their first point of contact. For people with less severe mental health problems (for example, anxiety), help will be offered at the primary care level. Larger fund-holding general practices often have their own attached counsellors and clinical psychologists to help with this sort of difficulty. The range of services likely to be available are:

- **advice and information**
- **prescribing**
- **counselling**
- **group therapy and family support.**

More severe problems, or those which do not respond to primary care interventions, are referred to specialist psychiatric services. This may be either the psychiatric out-patient clinic, or the community mental health team.

The Outpatient Clinic

The psychiatrist will see clients in the outpatient clinic. This can happen within a few days if the case is urgent although, more usually, there is a waiting time. If the problem is particularly urgent, the GP can ask the consultant psychiatrist to visit and assess the client at home. This is called a domiciliary visit or (DV). It is usually done within a day or two of the referral.

The Community Mental Health Team (CHMT)

A recent national survey identified that CMHTs are now a feature of mental health services in 96% of health authorities. The survey found that community psychiatric nurses and social workers were the most common CMHT members, but a proportion of teams also included psychologists, occupational therapists, doctors and support workers.

One multi-disciplinary mental health team will take on responsibility for a sector of usually between 20,000 and 30,000 population size. The sectors are usually defined by geographical boundaries, although there is now a move towards sectors being based on existing general practices and the population they serve. Both these models have advantages. The geographical sectorization allows closer relationships with geographically defined social services and the general practice based sectorization allows closer liaison with primary care services. Some CMHTs will also accept self-referrals.

Community mental health teams are responsible for supporting people with mental health problems and their carers who live in the community. The service users may either live in their own homes or in residential facilities. The teams undertake ongoing assessments and monitoring of the service users' mental health needs within the framework of the CPA and care management. **The sharing of information and effective communication are crucial to the role of the community mental health team.**

The roles of members of the mental health care team

Mental health problems often need a range of approaches. The mental health care team contains professionals with a wide variety of skills.

- **Psychiatric nurses** are based either in hospitals, including day hospitals, or else work mainly in the community as community psychiatric nurses. Individual community psychiatric nurses (CPNs) have caseloads of clients with serious mental illness, ideally less than 20 but often up to 50 or more. CPNs visit clients at home giving practical advice, helping with problems, often supervising medication and giving injections and helping with supportive counselling.

- **Occupational therapists** have skills based around helping clients to gain and strengthen abilities in daily living. These include a range of abilities, from basic day to day skills of cooking and cleaning to occupational and vocational skills training. The setting for this is often the day hospital or day centre.

- The **social worker** involved is usually an Approved Social Worker (ASW), meaning that they have had special mental health training and are approved to act under *The Mental Health Act, 1983*. The ASW targets the social needs of the client ensuring that he or she receives all the statutory benefits, arranging financial support if needed and liaising with a range of social services agencies such as housing services. ASWs have a range of counselling skills and may therefore become involved in interventions such as relationship work and family therapy. ASWs will be involved in assessments of mental health crisis when compulsory admission is being considered.

- **Mental health support workers** are a group of workers that have emerged over recent years as an important resource for working with people with serious and enduring mental illnesses living in the community. What differentiates their contribution from other groups of workers is a focus on the whole person in the social context and the use of a close and sustained relationship as the basis for help. While activity is frequently concentrated on aspects of daily living, this is done for the purpose of raising their client's confidence, self esteem and coping capacities, so as to minimise the damaging affects of remaining within the security of the "sick person role"

  Support workers are increasingly employed across the statutory, voluntary and private sectors. The notion of "support" primarily conveys the nature of their practice as opposed to their working relationship with other professional groups.

- The **clinical psychologist** involved has an undergraduate degree in psychology and a further postgraduate degree in clinical psychology. The clinical psychologists are particularly skilled in many forms of psychological treatment such as behaviour therapy, cognitive therapy and specific forms of counselling. Clinical psychologists

may be part of the mental health team or have a separate department within mental health services or be attached to GP surgeries.

- The **consultant psychiatrist** has a degree in medicine and at least 6 years training after that in psychiatry. He or she will have specialised either in adult psychiatry or in one of the sub-specialties such as child and adolescent psychiatry, old age psychiatry, learning disability or forensic psychiatry. Technically, he or she has a legal responsibility for medical treatment. As well as the consultant psychiatrist, there will usually be one or more junior psychiatrists in training attached to the team. These will either be basic registrars or a more senior specialist registrar (originally called senior registrars) who will have passed their professional exams set by the Royal College of Psychiatrists (MRCPsych). Psychiatrists are the only members of the team able to prescribe medication.

Urgent Cases

People in need of urgent psychiatric assessment may present to Accident and Emergency Departments, or be identified by the police, or at other points in the criminal justice system. In some authorities, diversion schemes may operate to ensure that people in the criminal justice system are identified and receive appropriate health and social services.

Some areas have developed "crisis intervention teams" as part of their mental health services. A team of workers will provide services in the home on an intensive basis, and aim to avoid hospital admission. Support to relatives and carers, as well as to the individual, will be provided.

If a mental health crisis cannot be managed in the community, compulsory admission under *The Mental Health Act, 1983,* may be necessary. (For a detailed discussion of *The Mental Health Act, 1983,* please refer to page 58).

Activity

Ask service users and colleagues to describe their experiences of mental health referral routes to the health and social services in your area.

SERVICES AND SETTINGS

Community Based Facilities for People with Mental Health Problems

A range of facilities are organised in the community by both social services and voluntary agencies - these include housing services, community centres for users and carers, welfare advice and employment schemes.

Community Residential Facilities

"Research demonstrates that provision of a suitable home is an important determinant of a mentally ill person's ability to live successfully in the community. Meeting this need will sometimes depend on the development of more specialised housing provision"[1].

The following are examples of the types of accommodation available for people with mental health problems and may be managed by either statutory, voluntary or independent providers.

- **Hospital Hostels** are designed to meet the needs of people with severely disabling long-term mental health problems. Nursing care is provided on a 24 hour basis and a close link with the hospital services is maintained. The hostels generally accommodate around 10 to 20 people. The first British hostel ward to be set up was 111 Denmark Hill, attached to the Maudsley Hospital,

London. The hostel's philosophy was that *"The unit was to be a house; a place for people to live in; but one where a high level of staffing facilities and supports - normally available only in a conventional hospital ward - would also be provided"*[2].

- **Hostels** are sometimes larger than hospital hostels (often accommodating 20 or more people) and are managed by either local authorities or voluntary organisations. They are regarded as short-term, rehabilitative, housing facilities with the aim of promoting the residents' independence. Staff employed in the hostels may include nurses, social workers and residential support workers. In some cases, 24 hour support is provided, in others, reduced staffing times are supplemented by an on-call system.

- **Supported Housing** schemes provide furnished accommodation for people with mental health problems who are able to live independently, but who appreciate the additional support of a housing support worker. The following is an example of the facilities which the Manchester based organisation, Creative Support, offers to residents in one of their supported housing projects

"Each person is allocated a support worker who visits whenever needed. Support workers work jointly with people in order to draw up an individual support plan. People are responsible for their own cooking and self care, but practical and emotional support can also be provided from a part-time support worker, dependent on individual needs."[3]

Other community residential facilities may include:

- Residential units provided by the voluntary, private and independent sector
- Therapeutic communities
- Registered mental nursing homes
- Long term residential care
- Respite residential care

Activity

Identify the range of residential facilities available for people with mental health problems in your area.

Community Based Support Facilities

A variety of facilities are available in the community including:

- A range of **educational and leisure services** is provided in most areas for use by the general public. People with mental health problems should be supported in using these facilities as appropriate to their interests and choices.

- **Day Centres** can be run by local authorities or the voluntary sector or by users themselves. A variety of activities are provided, many communal and some involving skill development (for example, computing, creative arts, and so on.)

- **Drop-in Centres** can be run by local authority or voluntary or user groups. They are available during the day and provide refreshments and some activities. They are often located in a building used by other community groups.

- **Carers' Centres** aim to provide support, information and advice to empower carers. Banbury Carers' Centre in North Oxfordshire has been set up to:

  - "provide information, advice and advocacy
  - reduce carers' isolation
  - offer carers a better choice of service
  - promote opportunities for carers to be involved in service planning, and in the development of the centre
  - work in partnership with other agencies"[4]

- **Employment Schemes** provide opportunities for people with mental health problems to work in environments which are both sympathetic to their individual needs and concerned with rehabilitation. Schemes are run by hospitals (industrial therapy), and by local authorities and communities.

Service Example
Turning Point, a nationwide organisation, run a project in Scotland, "PIP Crafts". The business is essentially run by business and craft personnel with mental health support. Funding for the project is mainly provided by the Mental Illness Specific Grant. The business produces a range of craft products which they sell to craft shops and fairs as well as to individuals. People who work for the organisation receive therapeutic earnings in the form of "top-up benefits". The main aims of the project are to:

- *Be run as a business, not a day centre;*
- *Create a working environment where people with mental health problems can gain skills whilst receiving additional support for their mental health needs;*
- *Develop artistic, craft and business skills;*
- *Teach workplace ethics, for example, punctuality.*

- **Welfare Rights Centres** offer advice and support on a range of financial, legal, employment and housing issues. The Citizens Advice Bureaux, Welfare Rights Units based in hospitals and social work departments offer these services. The Benefits Agency may also provide a specialist liaison worker. Typical queries dealt with might include advice on how to claim certain benefits, support in court cases, appeals and tribunals and assistance in dealing with housing problems. In some areas the voluntary sector organisations may also offer advice, for example, MIND.

Hospital Based Facilities for People with Mental Health Problems

The changes in the National Health Service since the mid - 1980s have seen the setting up of NHS Trusts in which an element of competition is assumed between different Trusts. Mental health facilities will either be managed within a larger NHS Trust, which includes all different types of medical and surgical specialties as well, or else in a separate mental health and community trust. Each of these two models has its advantages although many claim that mental health trusts allow the special needs of mental health to be focused on more clearly. A variety of well recognised hospital based facilities are likely to exist in the mental health services provided.

- **Day hospital** settings are usually on a District General Hospital site close to the acute inpatient unit. People with more severe, short lived problems can come up to the day hospital several times a week without needing to be admitted as inpatients. Some day hospitals also serve as a "staging post" for people recovering from a severe inpatient episode, on their way back into the community.

- **Outpatient clinics** will comprise adult psychiatry clinics, as well as specialist clinics such as old age and child psychiatry as well as psychotherapy, clinical psychology, psychosexual clinics and depot clinics (where people with schizophrenia and other disorders can receive depot injections).

- **Inpatient units** are much smaller than they once were and it is uncommon for a health district to have many more than 100 acute adult beds. People admitted to inpatient units are usually actively ill and the length of the stay varies a lot. It is typically 3 or 4 weeks. Most wards are open and free for patients to come and go. A minority, however, are secure or locked, often called intensive care units.

- All health districts will have access to some **intensive care unit** beds. These are for highly disturbed patients who need short term management, usually under *The Mental Health Act, 1983*. There are a range of other services such as eating disorder services, mother and baby units (for mothers with sudden mental health problems to be admitted along with their babies) and medium secure units for mentally disordered offenders.

● ●

DILEMMA

You have been informed that one of the members attending the mental health day centre where you work is described as exhibiting "attention seeking behaviour". He is extremely demanding of staff in the centre and has been disrupting the organised activities. He is not showing any signs of being violent. You have been advised to avoid giving him the attention he is after. He is, however, creating havoc in the centre and is disturbing other members.

What do you do?

The phrase "attention seeking behaviour" is overused and subjective.

- try to understand the behaviour being exhibited from the perspective of what you know about the person in the

past. Some users do exhibit attention seeking behaviour at times but this will be a repeating pattern in people usually with a history of personality problems. The notion underlying the concept of "attention seeking behaviour" is that it is completely under the control of the individual and that any sort of positive reinforcement will make it worse and more likely to occur in the future. Whereas this is certainly the case for true attention seeking behaviour, the risk is that other causes of disturbed behaviour are missed and not managed appropriately.

- Under all circumstances, unless there is a threat of physical violence, some attempt must be made to talk to the person, no matter how briefly. The two most common causes of "attention seeking behaviour" in day to day mental health practice are intoxication by drugs or alcohol and the reappearance of psychotic symptoms. Drug or alcohol intoxication may be fairly easy to detect, particularly if there is a previous history of this.

- Ask a key worker or another member of the team for information about the person's current state of mental health - re-emergence of psychotic phenomena is likely in someone with a history of schizophrenia or severe manic depression.

- Most day units will have a policy of excluding the person exhibiting the "attention seeking behaviour" and if that behaviour happens again they may decide to draw up a contract with the user.

- Remember to look after your own personal safety in situations like this. If someone is being disruptive, never try and interview them alone.

- If the disruption continues, then it may be necessary to exclude the person forcibly or call the police.

What other possible courses of action might you take?

(For further information on Managing Risk of Violence see Module 4)

● ●

TYPES OF INTERVENTION

WHAT TYPES OF PHYSICAL INTERVENTIONS ARE AVAILABLE?

A number of physical treatments including drug therapy and electro-convulsive therapy (ECT) are available to treat the symptoms of mental health problems. Whilst many people experience significant improvements with these treatments, they can have distressing side-effects in some. It is important that both the client and his or her relatives/carers understand fully how the treatment works, what to expect and the limitations of the treatment. **Physical intervention is not in itself a simple cure. The social and psychological dimensions of mental illness must also be addressed.**

DRUG TREATMENTS

Anxiolytics

This is the name given to a class of drugs which are given to lessen the symptoms of anxiety. Anxiety symptoms are usually a healthy response to the stresses of daily life and do not require medication. However, in some individuals, anxiety symptoms can be unusually severe and persistent and give rise to a generalized anxiety disorder or anxiety state. This may or may not include such features as panic attacks.

One avenue for treatment of severe anxiety symptoms is anxiolytic drugs. The most widely used type of anxiolytic drugs are still the **benzodiazepines**. This is a group of drugs which has been available since the 1960s and includes such examples as:

- diazepam (Valium),
- chlordiazepoxide (Librium), and
- lorazepam (Ativan).

By acting on the brain pathways that trigger anxiety, these drugs can be very effective over the short term. As a result they were widely prescribed in the 1970s and 1980s. However, their main drawback is that they are habit forming,

given over periods of longer than a few weeks and people prescribed benzodiazepines will start to need more to get the same effect. In addition, when people try to stop taking them, they will often experience unpleasant withdrawal effects such as rebound anxiety, insomnia and mood swings. As a result, benzodiazepines are prescribed less widely than they used to be and their prescription should be limited to relatively short periods. Psychological intervention such as cognitive behaviour therapy and anxiety management techniques are often preferred (these will be described later in this module).

Hypnotics

This is the name given to drugs which are similar to anxiolytics, but are given at night specifically to help sleep - they are more often called **sleeping tablets**. Those most often used have an overlap with the anxiolytic drugs in terms of their effects and side effects. Thus, they can be habit forming and should usually be used for a few weeks only at a time.

The most widely prescribed hypnotic is temazepam. This has recently become a street drug, sold on the black market. Anxiolytics and hypnotics are, despite their mild addictive qualities, fairly safe even if people take an intentional or accidental overdose.

As with anxiety, difficulty in sleeping is usually an understandable response to day to day stress. Common sense techniques such as avoiding cigarettes and alcohol in the evening, getting some physical exercise and having hot milky drinks before bed should, therefore, be tried first. Behavioural intervention may also be useful (this will be described later in this module).

Antipsychotic drugs

Other names given to this class of drugs are neuroleptic drugs and major tranquillizers. They all mean the same thing. These are drugs given to combat the acute symptoms of serious mental illness such as schizophrenia and severe mania. They don't act as straight sedatives but have a specific action on the part of thinking that creates delusions, hallucinations and thought disorder.

Antipsychotic drugs work in about 70% of people with psychotic symptoms of schizophrenia, but have a range of problems attached to them. They don't start working straight away and can take 2 or 3 weeks to have any effect. They don't work in about a third of people with schizophrenia.

Antipsychotic drugs are not habit forming, but they do have a range of side effects which many people will experience. The most common of these are problems with movement and this usually shows itself in a slowing down of facial expression and spontaneous body language. These are sometimes referred to as **extrapyramidal symptoms**. Although not dangerous, they can be upsetting and should be tackled either by reducing the dosage of the antipsychotic drug or by using a specific antidote to the side effects such as procyclidine (Kemadrin) tablets, a so-called anticholinergic drug.

Other side effects of antipsychotic drugs include unwanted sedation, particularly with drugs such as chlorpromazine (Largactil) and thioridazine (Melleril). Another (extrapyramidal) side-effect is akathisia, which is a strange subjective feeling of restlessness in the legs, often causing people to shuffle their legs constantly. This is under-recognized and can be an important cause of unexplained restlessness in people on antipsychotic drugs.

In the long term, an unusual but important side-effect is tardive dyskinesia, where the person develops involuntary movements of the mouth and face. Other rarer side-effects include jaundice, skin rashes, weight gain, sexual problems and heart problems in people with a history of heart disease.

Despite these side-effects antipsychotic drugs remain the first and most usual treatment for schizophrenia. Other commonly used anti-psychotic drugs are:

- haloperidol,
- trifluoperazine (Stelazine) and
- droperidol.

As well as being used to treat acute symptoms of schizophrenia, antipsychotic drugs are used to keep people well after they have recovered - **maintenance treatment**. Antipsychotic drugs, taken as maintenance treatment, are usually given in a smaller dose than for acute treatment.

Compliance can be a problem and this is understandable in that the drugs have side effects. People taking antipsychotic drugs need to be given a full explanation of the likely side effects and a full explanation of the benefits and then a risk - benefit decision can be made: do the benefits of preventing relapse outweigh the risks of side-effects, for instance?

Maintenance antipsychotic drug treatment can often be given in a once a day dose and is sometimes more convenient by syrup. An alternative is the use of depot antipsychotic medication which is given as an injection into the buttock, usually once a month. The most commonly used drugs are Depixol and Modecate. Once injected, the drug is released slowly over the next weeks. The main advantage of depot medication for the client is convenience. Disadvantages are a slightly increased risk of side-effects and some people find the monthly ritual of an injection painful and demeaning. Depot and anti-psychotic drugs can be given in hospital units and depot clinics by community psychiatric nurses, or in general practice surgeries.

Just as antipsychotic drugs can take a short period of time to start working, if a client stops his or her medication, the beneficial effects will last for several weeks before there is a risk of relapse. During this time clients may feel particularly well since they lose any side effects while still receiving the tail end of the beneficial effects.

In general terms, someone diagnosed as having schizophrenia stands about a 60% chance of relapsing within a year if he/she discontinues maintenance treatment with antipsychotic drugs, compared to about 10-20% of relapse if he/she takes medication. This is a generalization, in that some people have a good outcome from schizophrenia and some people will relapse even on medication.

Clozapine

This is an antipsychotic drug of a new type which has been available since 1990. It is unusual in that it causes none of the usual extrapyramidal side-effects. However, it does cause a group of side-effects of its own, the most serious of which is a rare but potentially fatal blood disorder. Despite this serious drawback, clozapine has been shown to be much more effective than any other antipsychotic drug in treating severe, persistent symptoms of schizophrenia. For about half such people, clozapine will significantly improve their quality of life. However, clients need to have regular (weekly to begin with) blood tests when taking clozapine to ensure they are not developing the blood disorder which occurs in less than 1% of people.

Clozapine is only prescribable for people with severe, persistent schizophrenia. It is expensive and many health authorities and trusts limit the number of people who can be given it. During 1997 and beyond, a new group of clozapine-like drugs which are safer will be appearing which may well replace many of the older drugs used in schizophrenia.

● ●

DILEMMA

Justin was diagnosed as having schizophrenia four years ago. He is now 25 and has not experienced symptoms of schizophrenia for the past 18 months. He is currently on a maintenance dose of an antipsychotic drug and feels that the time has come to try to come off his medication.

What do you do? What issues would you consider in giving him advice?

- Clarify why he is considering stopping the medication. Is he experiencing side effects such as tiredness, muscle stiffness or weight gain? Occasionally users attribute unrelated physical effects to their medication.

- Justin may believe that the medication is not doing him any good. This may be because the doctor who prescribed the medication did not explain adequately what the medication is intended to do. It would therefore be useful to clarify if Justin knows why he is taking the medication in the first place. In some instances, users may have delusions about the medication but far more usual is the existence of real reasons for wanting to stop, such as a lack of information or the experience of side effects.

- Ask Justin whether he has actually stopped the medication.

- Ask him if he has stopped in the past and what the consequences were.

- Point out that rather than stopping the medication altogether it may be that there is scope for reducing the dosage.

The ultimate decision of whether to stop the medication is Justin's and he should be urged to discuss this fully with the doctor who has prescribed the medication before making the decision. You should not, on establishing the facts, be drawn into finding yourself disagreeing with or confronting Justin.

Remember, all such decisions are based on a risk/benefit equation. Do the risks (such as side-effects) of taking the medication outweigh the benefits (protection against relapse for instance)?

No-one likes taking medication for long or indefinite periods and many aspects of wishing to stop medication can be viewed as signs of health rather than illness.

What other issues might you consider?

● ●

Antidepressants

This is a group of drugs which is different from the anxiolytics. They are not habit forming and do not lead to a withdrawal syndrome, unlike benzodiazapines. They are used mainly for moderate and severe depression although they can be effective in some people with severe anxiety as well.

As with anxiety, feeling depressed is usually a normal part of the day to day stresses of everyday life. However, some people are more vulnerable to prolonged and severe depression with insomnia, loss of appetite and weight and unalterable low mood day after day. Antidepressant drugs will work in about 70-80% of people with symptoms of severe depression.

In severe depression, the brain's arousal and biological rhythm centres become impaired. Antidepressant drugs set these body clock mechanisms back to normal by correcting brain substances such as serotonin (5HT). The older antidepressants are often called **tricyclic antidepressants** and include drugs such as:

- amitriptyline (Tryptizol),
- imipramine,
- clomipramine (Anafranil) and
- dothiepin (Prothiaden).

These drugs are usually taken in one daily dose in the evening. They take at least a week and up to 4 weeks to start working. The older tricyclic type antidepressants have side-effects. The most common of these is a dry mouth. In addition, some people, particularly older people experience:

- drowsiness,
- trembling,
- difficulty in passing urine, and
- giddiness and even blackouts when standing up quickly from being seated.

This last side-effect is due to the body not being able to correct normal drops in blood pressure. As well as these side effects, the older antidepressants can be dangerous, if taken in overdose, by producing heart problems.

Since the late 1980s, a range of newer antidepressants has become available with much fewer side effects. Also they are relatively safe, even if taken in overdose. Examples of safer antidepressants are lofepramine, as well as the so-called serotonin specific reuptake inhibitors (SSRIs) - the most well known of these is fluoxetine (Prozac). Other SSRIs include:

- fluvoxamine,
- sertraline and
- paroxatine.

When someone who is severely depressed gets better with antidepressants, they should usually expect to continue taking them for at least 6 months to avoid a relapse.

Antidepressants, such as SSRIs, can be surprisingly effective in some clients with other problems including bulimia (an eating disorder), obsessive compulsive disorders and some types of severe anxiety. In general, they are more effective with less concerns about addiction than the anxiolytic drugs.

Lithium

This is a mood stabilizing drug. It is extremely effective in most people who are diagnosed as having severe manic depression (bipolar disorder with depressed episodes and manic episodes). In most people with this disorder, lithium will prevent relapse if taken on a daily basis. However, there is, as always, a risk-benefit equation. Lithium has, potentially, very unpleasant side effects, if too much is taken, these include:

- nausea and vomiting,
- diarrhoea,
- trembling, and
- unsteadiness.

For this reason, clients taking lithium have 3 or 6 monthly blood tests to make sure that they are taking the right amount. The blood test measures the amount of lithium, and if this is too high, the dosage should be decreased. When taken in normal doses, lithium has few side effects.

ECT

ECT is electroconvulsive therapy, otherwise known as electric shock treatment. It is used much less widely than 20 years ago. Because it is an unpleasant sounding treatment, and because nobody quite knows how it works, its use should be kept to a minimum. Its use these days is really confined to clients with very severe depression, which has resisted other treatments - this is depression which is so severe that people develop delusions and hallucinations and stop eating and drinking. Although there is no doubt that ECT can work in extremely severe depression, the pros and cons should be fully discussed with the client.

The client is given a short-acting general anaesthetic which relaxes muscles and lasts about half an hour. While the person is asleep, he/she is made to have a fit which is exactly like an epileptic fit, but briefer. ECT is usually only given to people who are in hospital and happens usually twice weekly, between 6 and 12 times.

There is no evidence that ECT causes any sort of long-term brain damage, although the client may say his or her memory feels sluggish for a day or two afterwards. In addition, the client may complain of headaches, nausea and drowsiness. The risks associated with undergoing a general anaesthetic also apply to the ECT procedure, and the client should be made aware of this. People who have received ECT treatment have varying experiences of the procedure- whilst some people do not find it too distressing, others may feel devastated by the treatment.

WHAT TYPES OF PSYCHOLOGICAL INTERVENTIONS ARE AVAILABLE?

The physical treatments so far discussed identify ways of treating "symptoms", not necessarily underlying psychological problems. A variety of psychological treatments exist to help people with mental health problems. These interventions are available through the health services and are also provided by voluntary agencies and private practitioners.

Everyone with empathy and common sense can offer some sort of psychological support. The most basic level of psychological treatment is counselling. Supportive psychotherapy offers more structure and interpretation, and can be done by most specialist mental health workers. In-depth psychodynamic therapy is offered by specialist psychotherapists. Cognitive and behaviour therapy are based on psychological learning principles and are the basis of much of the work of clinical psychologists. As well as individual therapy, there is couple therapy, small group therapy and family therapy. It is important that individuals offering any kind of therapy should be appropriately trained and supervised.

Counselling

This involves the most basic elements that are common to all different sorts of psychological therapy. First of all it involves listening to the client. Often this will involve the client talking about ideas he or she has not put into words before. Restoring morale is an important part of counselling. Release of emotion can be helpful on occasions.

Counselling, like all forms of psychological treatment involves the setting up of a rationale or explanation that the client can use to make his or her problems more understandable. Counselling is usually planned over a relatively brief period of a few weeks. It also includes giving practical advice and ideas about problem solving for practical day to day issues. Counselling services are offered within the health service and by a number of voluntary organisations, for example, The Samaritans.

Supportive therapy

This is a more in-depth version of counselling. Again, the client is encouraged to talk about problems, while the therapist listens. The therapist's function often is to identify repeating patterns of behaviour and encourage the client to take responsibility for working out solutions collaboratively with the therapists. Careful and attentive listening is central to supportive therapy. It is important that the client feels he or she is being listened to and taken seriously.

Psychodynamic therapy

This is the sort of psychotherapy that is based on the more classical ideas of psychoanalysts such as Freud, Klein and Jung. Partly because it is usually long term, (at least once a week for a year or more) and partly because the evidence for its effectiveness is conflicting, psychodynamic therapy has become less widely available in the NHS, although it is still widely available in the private sector.

Using the theoretical models developed by Freud and his followers, the therapist attempts to discover unconscious thoughts and feelings which are claimed to be relevant to current difficulties. Concepts such as transference (development by the client of strong positive or negative feelings towards the therapist) and counter-transference (feelings the therapist gets about the client) are explored in detail.

This approach is of no practical use in serious mental illnesses such as schizophrenia and indeed can make the symptoms worse. Its main use is for long-standing neurotic personality problems, including those arising out of adverse childhood experiences. Less intense versions of psychodynamic therapy are often used in group therapy which have become increasingly common in helping people with neurotic and personality problems, including the victims of physical and sexual abuse in childhood.

Family therapy

This is mainly used where the client is an older child or adolescent. Family therapy can be useful for emotional or behaviour problems in adolescence, including anorexia nervosa and other eating disorders. Family therapists are generally skilled in working with families in this way.

Another version of family intervention has been increasingly used in schizophrenia. Although disturbed family life is not any longer thought to be the cause of schizophrenia, there is no doubt that family influences can make better or worse what happens to someone with schizophrenia, once he/she has developed it. Families with high degrees of distress, hostility and chaotic ways of managing problems (sometimes called **high expressed emotion** families) can precipitate relapse in someone with schizophrenia (for a further discussion of expressed emotion, refer to Module 1, page 12). With such families, it is often advisable either to suggest the client spends less time in face to face contact, or else to try and help the family find new ways of coping with day to day life.

Education as to the nature and symptoms of schizophrenia is an important first step, as is the trouble shooting of problem solving behaviour generally. Although these family interventions have been shown to be effective in reducing relapse rates in serious mental illnesses, they are still seldom applied in practice.

Group therapy

Groups are organised so as to deal with certain problems, (for example, a group for people with a diagnosis of schizophrenia), or with the development of certain skills, (for example, assertiveness training). Such a group situation provides the opportunity for its members to:

- share their experiences and learn from the experiences of others;

- gain support from people who have been through similar experiences;

- develop a feeling of belonging and respect as a member of a group who share their experiences, in order to help others;

- practice and develop social skills and gain confidence in relating to others.

- gain information, for example, practical information about the side effects of drugs and how to deal with them.

Such groups should be led by appropriately qualified staff.

Behaviour therapy

This is the name given to a set of techniques developed in the late 1950s and 60s to modify behaviour. In its clearest form, little or no account is taken of the thoughts and feelings underlying the behaviour. Behaviour therapy is mainly successful in disorders involving anxiety and some specific stimulus which triggers anxiety. Disorders which respond best to behaviour therapy are:

- phobias,
- psychosexual disorders, and
- obsessive compulsive disorders.

In treating straightforward phobias, the client is encouraged first to imagine and then actually to confront physically the feared stimulus, be it spiders, heights or open spaces. A similar strategy is used in obsessive-compulsive disorders, where the client again is exposed to the stimulus which will trigger his/her compulsive ritual, such as hand washing or checking.

By using step by step graded exposure to increasing the anxiety provoking version of the stimulus (first an imagined spider, then a picture of a spider, then a model of a spider, then a real spider) the client will learn to habituate to the stimulus and the anxiety will gradually wear off. For fairly straightforward phobias, these techniques are usually successful.

Cognitive therapy

Cognitive therapy, or cognitive behaviour therapy, is a more recent development. It takes as its starting point that in disorders such as anxiety and depression, clients will often develop patterns of thinking that are wrong or inappropriate. In anxiety management, clients are helped to recognise intrusive, unwanted thoughts which precipitate anxiety. They can then be taught to distract themselves from these thoughts, or to repeat to themselves rational statements which make the thoughts go away.

In depression, people often develop negative patterns of thinking, drawing negative conclusions from everyday neutral events. In this way ideas of self-blame, low self-esteem, guilt and hopelessness develop. In cognitive therapy for depression, the recurrence of intrusive thoughts is again monitored and interrupted by distraction or self-reassurance. Irrational patterns of thinking are identified and alternative explanations given.

Cognitive therapy is essentially a collaborative technique, usually given by a clinical psychologist. It usually involves homework for the client and keeping diaries of thoughts, feelings and actions.

All the available evidence suggests that cognitive behaviour therapy outperforms counselling and simple and psychodynamic psychotherapy for most anxiety and depression related mental health problems. Most recently, a variation of cognitive therapy has been used partly successfully in schizophrenia as an adjunct to, but not an alternative to drug treatment. The next few years may see an increased use of cognitive therapy in this area.

Activity

If a service user asked for advice on how to select a private/voluntary sector counsellor in your area, what issues might you consider?

- Which direction would you point them in for further advice?

References

1 Department of Health. *The Spectrum of Care. Local Services for People with Mental Health Problems.* London: Department of Health.

2 Philippa Garety (1991) *Residential Needs for Severely Disabled Psychiatric Patients - The Case for Hospital Hostels.* London: HMSO.

3 Creative Support (1996) *Supported Accommodation - Project Leaflet.*

4 Social Services Inspectorate (1995) *What Next for Carers?* London: SSI.

Recommended Reading

Goldberg D., Benjamin S. and Creed F. (1994) *Psychiatry in Medical Practice.* 2nd edition. London: Routledge.

Onyett, S., Heppleston, T. and Bushnell, D. (1994) *The organisation and operation of community mental health teams in England.* London: The Sainsbury Centre.

Onyett S., Pillinger T. and Muijen M. (1995). *Making Community Mental Health Teams Work: CMHTs and the people who work in them.* London: Sainsbury Centre for Mental Health.

Morgan S. (1993) *Community Mental Health.* London: Chapman & Hall.

• •

This module - "Intervention and Management" - is one of 7 modules in "Learning Materials on Mental Health - an Introduction". The other modules include:

Module 1 - "Recognition of Mental Health Problems"

Module 3 - "Legislation and Guidance"

Module 4 - "Special Client Groups"

Module 5 - "Special Issues"

Module 6 - "Users, Carers and Children of Parents with Mental Health Problems"

Module 7 - "Sample Training Exercises"

A sister set of materials is also available for professionals involved in assessing risk - " Learning Materials on Mental Health Risk Assessment"

module 3

LEGISLATION AND GUIDANCE

AIMS & OBJECTIVES

After you have worked through this module you should be better able to:

- Discuss the impact which recent health and social care legislation has had on mental health services.

- Describe the principles of the Care Programme Approach.

- Summarise the functions of *The Mental Health Act, 1983*.

- Describe the provisions of other mental health legislation.

THE FRAMEWORK FOR PROVIDING MENTAL HEALTH SERVICES

Mental health services have undergone significant changes since the late 1980s. Changes in the law and in guidance from government have inevitably reflected the thinking of politicians on the role, structure and operation of the public sector as well as changing philosphies of service.

This module summarises legislation and central government guidance most relevant to enabling services to be provided for people with mental health problems and, in some cases, other people who need help and special services. Services are provided by local authority social services departments, health authorities and independent providers.

The relevant legislation and guidance is summarised below in date order.

THE MENTAL HEALTH ACT, 1983 AND THE CODE OF PRACTICE, 1993

This Act establishes the framework for the compulsory admission of people to psychiatric hospitals and covers a range of provisions in relation to detained patients. When a person has symptoms of mental disorder which cannot be managed in the usual social setting, compulsory admission can be a consideration. Individuals may be admitted under Section 2 of the Act for assessment (28 days maximum), Section 3 for treatment (6 months maximum), and under Section 4 in situations of urgent necessity (72 hours maximum). The need for detention has to be in the interests of the person's health or safety, or for the protection of other people. *The Code of Practice*, 1993 gives guidance on the application of *The Mental Health Act, 1983* and clarifies the roles of the professionals involved.

The Mental Health Act, 1983, confers a statutory role on the Approved Social Worker (ASW), who must apply for compulsory detention in situations where "he is satisfied such application ought to be made..." (S.13(1)). This is an

independent decision resting on the ASW's professional judgement, though generally involving close collaboration with psychiatric colleagues and supervision from experienced senior staff. Applications must be supported by two medical recommendations (one in urgent situations). The role of the ASW in decision-making when compulsory detention is being considered is unique to the UK, and brings an element of social assessment as well as psychiatric assessment to situations of mental health crisis. The Act stipulates that social workers who seek to become approved by their employing local authorities have to have "appropriate competence in dealing with persons who are suffering from mental disorder" (S.114(2)), and that local authorities must appoint sufficient ASWs to fulfill duties under the Act (S.114(1)).

Case example of a person admitted under The Mental Health Act, 1983: Barry

Barry Horton, who was described in Module 1(p. 8) and Module 2(p. 41), is being supported with a package of care under the Care Programme Approach. This includes a place at a local day centre. A worker at the day centre contacts the key worker Clive, to tell him that Barry feels he no longer needs his medication. The key worker, who is a CPN, is aware that Barry missed his last injection a week ago. Both have tried to explain to Barry the importance of taking his medication regularly.

Clive visits Barry at home regularly and keeps in touch with Barry's parents with whom he is living. His parents report that his behaviour at home is deteriorating. He is becoming very withdrawn, seldom leaving his room during the day, his hygiene is becoming poor, and he is increasingly abusive and threatening towards his parents. His mother says he has started talking to himself again.

Clive arranges a Care Programme Review meeting because of the changes in Barry and the anxieties expressed by his parents. The team agree that Barry needs treatment, but Barry refuses any and will not come into hospital. The psychiatrist and the Approved Social Worker agree to meet the GP at his surgery. The GP visited Barry's home the previous day and says that Barry was agitated and hallucinating. When the Psychiatrist and the ASW visit Barry, he has the same symptoms, and is adamant that he needs no treatment. An application under Section 3 of The Mental Health Act, 1983, is made by the ASW. Barry is admitted to hospital.

Part 3 of the Act is concerned with people experiencing mental disorders who are involved in criminal proceedings or under sentence of the courts. Sections 35 and 36 enable people appearing before the courts on criminal charges to be remanded to hospital for a report on their mental condition or for treatment for a mental illness or severe mental impairment. Section 37 enables courts to make an order authorising detention in hospital, or placing the individual under a guardianship order, following a conviction normally resulting in imprisonment (subject to specified conditions). Section 41 of the Act provides for the imposition of a "restriction order" when a hospital order is made. When patients are restricted, they may be discharged only by the Home Secretary or a Mental Health Review Tribunal. Patients may be discharged (section 42) subject to conditions which may include supervision by a psychiatrist, social worker or probation officer. Social supervisors are required to keep in regular contact with discharged restricted patients.

Prisoners may be transferred to psychiatric hospitals under specified conditions in *The Mental Health Act, 1983* (Sections 47, 48 and 49).

Other provisions of *The Mental Health Act, 1983,* include rights of appeal to Mental Health Review Tribunals, provisions for consent to treatment, the functions of nearest relatives and the management of the property and affairs of patients by the Court of Protection.

Whilst *The Mental Health Act, 1983,* is generally seen as the framework governing detained patients, it also contains important sections which have a bearing on continuing care in the community. Sections 7 and 8 of the Act describe the

conditions under which an application for guardianship may be made to the local authority. These are similar to those for a compulsory admission under Section 3. Guardianship gives specific powers to those acting as Guardians:

* the power to require the individual to live in a specific place;

* the power to require the person to attend for medical treatment, occupation, education or training.

* the power to require access to the person by a doctor, social worker or any other specified person.

Guardianship has been little used, being seen as lacking in powers of enforcement (for example, it does not give the right to coerce or convey). There are, inevitably, resource implications, which fall on local authorities if it is used frequently. Current debates on supervision in the community mirror the dilemmas of its use.

Section 117 of the Act requires health and local authorities to provide aftercare services for certain patients discharged from psychiatric hospitals until those services are no longer needed. People who have been detained under Sections 3, 37, 47 and 48 are included - these are the longer-term detention provisions and include people who have entered psychiatric care via the courts. The implementation of Section 117 has been patchy and unsystematic for many years, but attention to its provisions has grown in recent years as other frameworks for the support of mentally ill people in the community have developed. Whilst people entitled to Section 117 services should also fall within the provisions of the care programme, it remains as an independent statutory right for the named categories of discharged patients.

THE CHILDREN ACT, 1989

This addresses the whole range of legislation in relation to the care of children, integrating existing law with new provisions. The Act's central principle is that in all legal decisions about the care of children, the welfare of the child shall be the paramount consideration. Local authorities also have a duty under the Act to support families in bringing up their children if this is consistent with the child's welfare.

The term "children in need" is used to describe children who need services in order to secure or maintain a reasonable standard of health and development (children with disabilities are included in the concept of "children in need"). As part of the support to families of "children in need", the Act authorises the provision of day-care services for pre-school children and supervised activities for school-age children after school hours or during holidays.

These powers offer scope for a much wider range of facilities than was possible under previous children's legislation. In identifying the principles of good child care practice, the Department of Health states;

"Even though services may be offered primarily on behalf of their children, parents are entitled to help and consideration in their own right. Just as some young people are more vulnerable than others, so are some mothers and fathers. Their parenting capacity may be limited temporarily or permanently by poverty, racism, poor housing or unemployment or by personal or marital problems, sensory or physical disability, mental illness or past life experiences."[1]

Local authorities are clearly empowered to provide services for children who are in families that are vulnerable due to parental mental illness, within their resource limits.

The Children Act, 1989, also contains the legal provisions under which abused or neglected children can be assessed without parental agreement, or can be removed from parental care and looked after by the local authority. In cases of alleged abuse or neglect, authorities are required to explore all options before resorting to compulsory powers. In some cases, parents who abuse or neglect their children may also have mental health problems.

Careful joint assessment and planning are essential in such cases to ensure that the needs of both parents and children are considered. Professionals whose primary concern is the mental health of adults should be fully aware that the welfare of any children must be evaluated as an issue in its own right. Parental mental ill-health can never be allowed to justify allowing the care of children to fall below an acceptable threshold.

CARING FOR PEOPLE, 1989

This White Paper describes how local authority social services departments organise and provide services for adult groups including people with physical, sensory or learning disabilities, as well as those with a mental illness. Its overall purpose was to promote a range of community care services to enable vulnerable people to live in the community, wherever possible. A further aim was to promote the development of a mixed economy of care.

Given that most adults needing social care services cannot pay the real cost, the White Paper stated that services would be allocated following an assessment of need. The main impetus for the White Paper, and the subsequent *NHS and Community Care Act, 1990*, sprang from a need to do something about the substantial growth in demand on the social security budget resulting from the increasing use of private residential care for older people. At that time, this was paid for automatically if the older person had no independent means.

The key objectives stated in Caring for People, 1989, are:

- to promote the development of domiciliary, day and respite services to enable people to live in their own homes whenever feasible and sensible

- to ensure that service providers make practical support for carers a high priority

- to make proper assessment of need and good care management the cornerstone of high quality care

- to promote the development of a flourishing independent sector alongside good quality public services

- to clarify the responsibilities of agencies and make it easier to hold them to account for their performance

- to secure better value for taxpayers' money by introducing a new funding structure for social care.

MENTAL HEALTH SERVICES FRAMEWORKS FOR PEOPLE ADMITTED INTO HOSPITAL AND DISCHARGED INTO THE COMMUNITY

Potential Pathways of Services for People Originally Admitted into Hospital on an Informal Basis

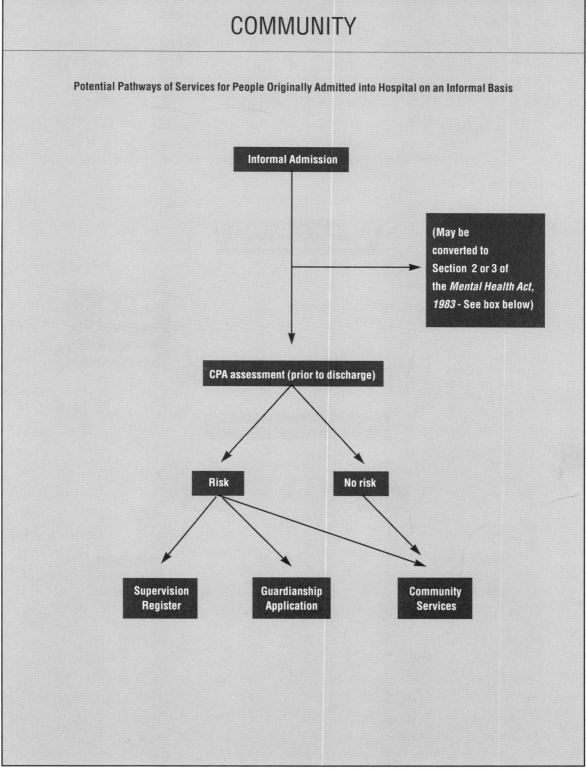

MENTAL HEALTH SERVICES FRAMEWORKS FOR PEOPLE ADMITTED INTO HOSPITAL AND DISCHARGED INTO THE COMMUNITY

People admitted formally into hospital under section 2 and 3 of the *Mental Health Act, 1983,* may appeal to tribunals or the hospital managers. Upon discharge into the community all patients are eligible for needs assessment via social services care management.

Potential Pathways of Services for People Originally Admitted into Hospital under Section 2 of the *Mental Health Act, 1983*

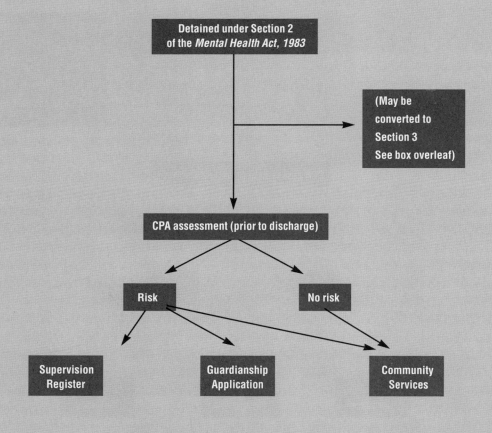

MODULE 3

MENTAL HEALTH SERVICES FRAMEWORKS FOR PEOPLE ADMITTED INTO HOSPITAL AND DISCHARGED INTO THE COMMUNITY

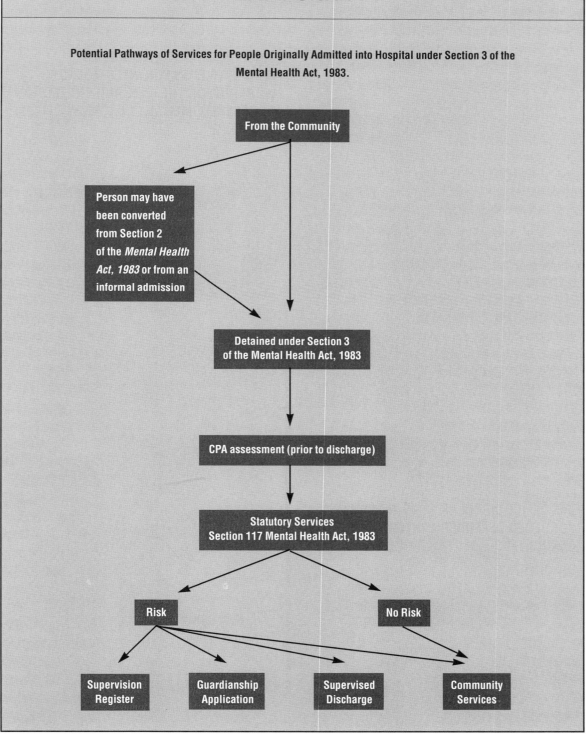

Potential Pathways of Services for People Originally Admitted into Hospital under Section 3 of the Mental Health Act, 1983.

From the Community

Person may have been converted from Section 2 of the *Mental Health Act, 1983* or from an informal admission

Detained under Section 3 of the Mental Health Act, 1983

CPA assessment (prior to discharge)

Statutory Services Section 117 Mental Health Act, 1983

Risk

No Risk

Supervision Register

Guardianship Application

Supervised Discharge

Community Services

CARERS (RECOGNITION AND SERVICES) ACT, 1995

This legislation applies to all informal carers of people assessed under the framework of *The NHS and Community Care Act, 1990*. The carer must provide a "substantial amount of care on a regular basis" for the person whose needs are being assessed. The 1995 Act states that the carer may ask the local authority to assess his/her ability to carry on providing care. The local authority has to take account of this assessment before making a decision on providing services.

This Act, whilst not bringing an increase in community care resources, serves to emphasise the position of informal carers of people with longer term disabilities. The impact of a carer's responsibilities have been well documented[2] yet they remain the primary resource for those needing longer term care - including people with mental health problems.

This legislation is not alone in addressing carers' needs. *The Disabled Persons (Services, Consultation and Representation) Act, 1986*, was the first to instruct local authorities to "have regard" to the abilities of carers to continue in their role, when assessing someone with a disability (Section 8).

The guidance to *The Carer's Act, 1995* asks authorities to take account of carers' individual circumstances and the support available to them in making assessments. Authorities should not assume a willingness to continue caring. Carers who are children or young people under 18 should be assessed in relation to their own developmental needs, and in relation to service provision under *The Children Act, 1989*.

HOME OFFICE CIRCULAR 12/95: MENTALLY DISORDERED OFFENDERS: INTER-AGENCY WORKING 1995

This circular endorses the basic principles of *The Reed Report, 1992* and summarises the progress of schemes receiving funding. It advocates "active cooperation" between the relevant agencies and the sharing of information in relation to an individual's current and past offending behaviour. All agencies, including the Crown Prosecution Service, are asked to balance considerations of the individual's mental health, as well as those of public safety, in

decisions relating to mentally disordered people in the criminal justice process. These include decisions on whether to charge, as well as decisions of the courts.

The circular endorsed the principle of "diversion" from the Criminal Justice System detailed in an earlier Circular (Home Office Circular 66/90).

BUILDING BRIDGES: A GUIDE TO ARRANGEMENTS FOR INTER-AGENCY WORKING FOR THE CARE AND PROTECTION OF SEVERELY MENTALLY ILL PEOPLE (1995)

This guide is published by the Department of Health within the broad strategy of *The Health of the Nation, 1992*. It's aim is "to promote close and effective inter-agency working so that well coordinated care can be delivered" (p.8). It also reaffirms Government policy that specialist mental health services target their resources upon those with severe mental illnesses as a priority.

The guide suggests a working definition of severe mental illness which includes five dimensions:

- **Diagnosis:** people experiencing some sort of mental illness (typically people diagnosed as having schizophrenia or a severe mood disorder, but including dementia);

- **Disability:** people who experience substantial disability as a result of their illness, such as an inability to care for themselves independently, sustain relationships or work;

- **Duration:** people who have current florid symptoms or have a chronic enduring condition (overall for periods of 6 months or more);

- **Informal or formal care:** people who have recurrent crises leading to frequent admissions or interventions (breakdown of informal and formal care delivered for usual support);

- **Safety:** people whose behaviour is a significant risk to themselves or others.

Not all of these conditions are necessary for a person to be regarded as severely mentally ill. Local health and social services authorities will develop their own operational criteria consistent with the definition in the guidance.

Building Bridges, 1995, provides a detailed summary of the frameworks for mental health service provision, and the working of the CPA and *The NHS and Community Care Act, 1990*. Its central theme is the importance of good inter-agency working in delivering complex service packages to severely disabled people.

KEY THEMES IN POLICY AND SERVICE PROVISION IN MENTAL HEALTH

Our analysis so far shows the key themes in the changes in service provision in the decade to 1996. These reflect changes in the philosophies underlying public service provision. We examine some of these themes and their implications for people with mental health problems in the following sections.

THE EFFICIENT TARGETING OF MENTAL HEALTH SERVICES

Service development has taken place against a background of economic recession and cuts in public expenditure. At the same time, reliance on psychiatric hospitals has diminished for economic and social reasons as well as advances in drug treatments. The number of psychiatric beds available nationally in the 1990s is less than a third of the peak number in the 1950s[3] and it is generally acknowledged that, except in extreme cases, people with mental health difficulties are better living in community settings.

The decrease in psychiatric beds has continued, irrespective of governments and through periods of economic growth as well as decline. It has been a phenomenon throughout the developed world and signals fundamental shifts in the attitudes of both public and professionals. People with mental health difficulties are no longer viewed as representing a problem to be hidden from view, but as a vulnerable group with rights and needs. Increasingly, services are geared to support them in their social context and outside hospital. Hospital admission may be used to deal with episodes which cannot otherwise be treated, or which involve high levels of risk.

The decline in psychiatric hospital provision through the 1970s and 1980s was achieved to a great extent through resettlement. Former "long-stay" patients were rehabilitated in the community, whilst their potential replacements - people with newly diagnosed severe psychiatric illnesses - were rarely admitted on a permanent basis. There is evidence that much of this rehabilitative work was successful in enabling people with lengthy hospital "careers" to establish themselves in the community[4]. People now diagnosed as having the more severe mental disorders - sometimes referred to as the "new long-stay" group, because they would formerly have become long-stay hospital patients - can experience periodic mental health crises. In addition, their daily lives in the community can require considerable support. Others may experience acute mental health crises from which they recover, but which makes a short-term demand on services. A spectrum of flexible services is, therefore, necessary to meet their needs. Recent government guidelines have emphasised that this spectrum must cater appropriately for those who need 24-hour nursing care. Concern is expressed that health authorities have not made adequate provision for the "new long-stay" group whose needs are such that 24-hour accommodation with supervision of medication and continuous monitoring of mental state is necessary[5].

We have seen a sustained policy towards better managed and targeted services in order to ensure that, despite limited resources, existing services are used to meet the most serious needs in the most effective ways. We have learned lessons from previous decades, in which a concern to make services easily accessible led to their being used mostly by those less severely disabled by mental illness. In the USA, community mental health centres operated on the principle of walk-in help, until it was acknowledged that those with severe and enduring mental illnesses are less likely to seek the help they may need[6]. As a result, service uptake may become skewed towards those whose problems are less severe.

Health of the Nation estimates of the prevalence of mental illnesses in the UK show that for every individual with schizophrenia there are roughly 10 with identified clinical depression; for every individual with affective psychosis there are 12 or more with anxiety related disorders[7]. Guidance in relation to *The Health of the Nation, 1992*, the Care Programme Approach and systems of care management in local authorities indicates a need to focus specialist psychiatric services on those with the most severe and disabling mental health problems. This may mean delivering services on an assertive basis, that is to people who might not come forward for help. Thought needs to be given to what makes a service attractive to people with severe disability and long term needs.

Health service guidance HSG(94)27 instructs NHS professionals and provider unit managers to "establish local guidelines, agreed with purchasers, to ensure that the necessary priority is given to meeting the needs of the most seriously ill patients". However, advice in *Building Bridges, 1995,* cautions against diagnosis being the sole criterion of severity, and suggests a number of examples of useful definitions[8]. These include the dimensions of diagnosis, disability, duration of illness, safety and formal and informal care and support.

Professionals working in the specialist services in hospitals and in the community are now under pressure to prioritise their time and resources in order to meet the needs of those most disabled by mental illness. An Audit Commission report published in 1994 indicated that specialist social workers in many districts were more likely to have higher proportions of severely mentally ill people on their caseloads than were community psychiatric nurses[9]. This may be tied up with the issue of access to the resources of care management in local authorities as they too, target the most severely disabled.

Our own experience suggests that it is sometimes those in support teams or rehabilitation teams who carry the caseloads with the highest proportion of severely ill people. However, this may be appropriate if supportive work is needed, provided that levels of complexity and risk are monitored and that specialised help from psychiatrists or suitably qualified staff is available[10].

Where the Care Programme Approach is implemented fully there should be an assessment of need for all those in contact with the specialist services or discharged from psychiatric hospital units. People with a high level of need should have continuity of support from a key worker. In some districts this is happening; in others arrangements are taking time to become established or resources are stretched and not everyone can be allocated a key worker. The careful management of provider services in both health districts and local authorities is necessary to ensure that individuals who are identified as having high priority receive the appropriate services.

One risk of targeting resources at the group with severe and enduring mental illness is that the needs of other groups are less likely to be met, for example, those with "less severe" mental health problems, such as depression and anxiety, and those with severe mental illness which does not become long term. This group of people is now seen as more appropriately helped by non-specialised services, delivered at primary care level[11], with perhaps more specialised support in periods of crisis.

Serious levels of distress still accompany all mental ill-health and there is likely to be a need for personal and social support. In the group with mental health problems described as "less severe" there is likely to be an over-representation of women with young children, and of older people, both groups being particularly vulnerable to depression[12,13]. The additional social vulnerability due to age/life stage and caring responsibilites adds weight to the need for support. Attempts are being made to raise the awareness of General Practitioners and other primary care staff about the recognition and response to mental health problems - the *Defeat Depression Campaign*[14] is an example of this approach.

A PERSON WITH A MENTAL HEALTH PROBLEM TREATED AT GP LEVEL: DIANE

Diane (42 years) visits her GP saying she is exhausted and at the end of her tether. Diane is married with three children aged 15, 11 and 7. Her husband has a small business which is struggling financially and he works long hours. Diane has to work to provide enough to cover the mortgage and other needs. She is a qualified nurse and works full-time at a hospital a few miles away. Child care has proved difficult to find, and Diane is worried about the effect on the youngest child of a number of changes.

Diane is responsible for all of the domestic tasks. She describes her husband as supportive, but stressed and over-worked. She feels she is in a "bottomless pit" and has had episodes of crying and shaking at work and is too tense to sleep. She feels unable to carry on, but cannot see any solution to the problems.

The GP sees Diane fortnightly, and prescribes anti-depressants. She gives Diane a sick note. She also arranges for Diane to see a counsellor employed at the GP practice. The counsellor explores with Diane and her husband possible changes they can make to relieve Diane of some of the continuing stress.

The GP also puts Diane in touch with a women's group run locally for women who experience depression. Here Diane is able to discuss the experience of depression and ways of managing it. Diane and her husband are able to agree some changes in their lives. She returns to work. The GP maintains monthly contact and advises continuing the medication.

This case illustrates how someone with depression can be helped at primary care level, using a range of resources. These will vary in their availability, and each client is likely to need an individualised response. Diane was able to cease medication after about 6 months and to take decisions which relieved some of the stress.

THE CONTROL OF QUALITY IN THE DELIVERY OF HEALTH AND SOCIAL SERVICES

The fundamental changes in the structure and funding of health and social services were intended to create a "quasi-market", within which the power of the consumer to make choices about spending would create competition between provider agencies in relation to quality and costs. Rather as if they were buying a car or any other consumer item, those with purchasing power would make choices and this, in turn, prompts the provider to become more competitive and efficient.

At its simplest this mechanism satisfies the twin aims of ensuring efficiency in providing and managing services, and matching individual need and service provided. Two issues complicate the simple market analogy. Firstly, providing

services for vulnerable adults is, for the most part, paid for out of the public purse. Therefore, the "consumer" is in reality a public purchasing organisation. Secondly, the commodity being bought is not an off-the-shelf product that can be evaluated by anyone, but a service that usually relies on the judgement of a trained professional in establishing need.

This is particularly so in the field of mental health, where the judgement of the consumer may be affected by illness. At times, services may be delivered that the individual concerned does not even want (for example, compulsory admission or treatment under *The Mental Health Act, 1983*).

Control of quality in health and social services is not safeguarded by the usual market mechanisms, but is mediated by purchaser organisations judging value-for-money and by professionals judging need and eligibility. At the level of purchasing, health and social services authorities can impose quality control by the mechanisms of contracting and service specification.

The Patients Charter[15] requires that detailed information be available about health services, including quality standards to be expected. Health authorities have to implement complaints procedures which offer the complainant an investigation and a reply. A charter specifically for mental health services is due to be published. In social services the mechanisms for controlling quality include complaints procedures and the duty to establish inspection of provider services. However, the statutory duty imposed on social services authorities by *The NHS and Community Care Act, 1990,* is to assess need but not necessarily to provide services to meet that need. Resource limits sometimes restrict the amount of service delivered.

The involvement of service users, carers and their service user and carer organisations in the planning and delivery of services is now an established principle in both the health and social services. This involvement at more than one level is another means of ensuring quality and the sensitivity of services for the consumer.

The principle is not only embedded into health and social care provisions for adults, but is also important in *The Children Act, 1989*. Even where there are issues of child protection, the rights of parents (or carers) to be consulted and have their views taken into account are still safeguarded. Children also have the right to be involved in decisions about themselves, depending on their age and level of understanding.

(Issues to do with service user and carer involvement are examined in more detail in Module 6).

Activity

- Find out the procedures and mechanisms for dealing with complaints about services provided within care management arrangements in your authority.
- How are service users and carers told about the procedures?

MULTI-DISCIPLINARY APPROACHES

Our approach to understanding mental health problems rests on the basic assumption that mental health difficulties are caused by a variety of factors in complex interaction. These range from biological and genetic factors, through individual psychology and couple or family dynamics, to pressures from the wider social, political and economic environment. Some specific mental health problems have been identified as having a more powerful biological component in their aetiology, whilst others may be the product more of life events, social stress or the limited psychological resilience of individuals.

All mental health problems have profound consequences for the well-being of the individual, not just in health terms but also in affecting interpersonal relationships, and roles and relationships in the wider social environment. The diversity of causes and consequences of mental ill health supports an approach to intervention which offers the potential of choice and "match" of the professionals involved in the person's care and support.

Current guidance emphasises the importance of multi-disciplinary and inter-agency work in community mental health services. In the CPA and care management frameworks, however, the identification of particular disciplines is avoided for key workers or care managers. Mental health professionals are encouraged to be organised

within community mental health teams[16] with care management and the Care Programme being integrated so that service users experience planned and continuous care.

The Care Programme Approach was developed for situations in which often highly vulnerable people drifted between services, with no one service or professional accepting core responsibility for their wellbeing. Fundamental to this was the responsibility of hospital-based services, once the person had been discharged. Planning for discharge and ongoing support are now the responsibility jointly of the psychiatrist, the clinical team and the community teams of health and social services staff[17]. Once discharged, vulnerable people should remain a team responsibility, with periodic reassessment of their needs and flexible access to a range of professional skills.

The role of the NHS in the continuing care of all those with long term health needs (including people with mental illnesses) has been clarified further in Circular HSG (95)8/LAC (95)5. The circular confirms that there is no automatic right to occupy a hospital bed in cases where there is no need for continuing NHS care, and that alternative arrangements can be made in the person's own home or in the community for those with long term needs.

The circular also makes clear that it is the responsibility of the NHS to arrange and fund a range of services, including support for health needs in the community, for those with long term needs who are not in hospital. This reaffirms the role of the NHS beyond hospital care. In the case of those with mental health needs, the approach supports the CPA framework.

The case of Christopher Clunis[18] highlights how an individual could move through a wide range of consecutive services, which had little coordination of care or information. Clunis was offered repeated out-patient appointments, but failed to use them. Hospital services felt that they had reached the limits of their responsibility. He was in contact with many community-based services, including social services and a range of housing agencies. Each agency tried to help, but no-one felt it their responsibility to record the history of help as Clunis moved from one area to another. Indeed, there were no mechanisms for doing so. A later case of S.L. again shows hospital-based services failing to maintain continuing responsibility for a discharged patient, despite the introduction of the Care Programme Approach in the interim period[19].

One of the issues underlying the organisation of multi-disciplinary work is that of the health and social care divide. Health authorities have statutory responsibility for health needs, since the NHS is based on the principle of a universal service free at the point of delivery. Social services authorities, on the other hand, have a range of statutory powers and duties concerning social and welfare needs. *The NHS and Community Care Act, 1990,* introduced the issue of costing and charging for these services, which are offered only on the basis of a needs assessment.

Adults with mental health difficulties are one of the groups whose needs for service are not easy to classify into either health or social care: mental illness has substantial social implications which generate a need for supportive services. However, it is far from clear whose responsibility it is to provide services which address these needs. A recent circular[20] required health authorities to produce local policies and eligibility criteria for continuing health care needs, agreed with social services departments and GP fundholders by April 1996. This should further clarify the role of the NHS in cases of long term health need.

The other complicating factor is the purchaser/provider split in the organisation of health and social services. In health services, the hospitals have been separated out as provider units and almost all have moved into independent trust status. NHS commissioning units operate in the purchasing role, hold budgets and negotiate contracts with providers. Fund-holding GPs operate as both purchasers and providers, but other "hands-on" community professionals are solely providers. This includes community psychiatric nurses and other community staff working with mentally ill people.

In social services departments, the purchaser/provider split is less clear cut, as the front-line services are supervised through the same lines of management across which the split operates (the senior managers act as heads of purchasing and are also managerially accountable for the services provided by the social services departments). In some departments, qualified social work staff have been designated as purchasers/assessors, whose primary role is not seen to

be one of front-line service delivery. Provider services include day or residential care units, support teams, or other elements of direct service.

The process of "care management" is the arranging (including costing and purchasing) of services to meet an individual's needs. One of the aims of separating assessment from provision is to make explicit the unit cost of services, enabling more informed decisions to be made about the management of resources within the mixed economy of care.

Activity

- Identify a service user who receives a "care package" of services within care management arrangements.
- Talk to the care manager about how the services are costed and purchased.
- Try and work out the cost of the individual package.

In some authorities, the impact of the new arrangements, as far as qualified social work staff are concerned, has been to emphasise the assessment component of their work and to reduce their role in providing direct service. In mental health social work, specifically trained ASWs are appointed under *the 1983 Mental Health Act.* In addition to making application for compulsory detentions, the *Mental Health Act Code of Practice, 1993*, advises a wider role for ASWs in providing a direct service to people assessed under the Act.

There are, therefore, differing implications for the ASW's role in providing a direct supportive or therapeutic service. Many authorities are approaching this in a practical way, deploying qualified mental health social workers to provide a direct service where there are high levels of risk or more complex or changing needs, but also to act as assessors under care management arrangements. Overall, "helping" has become less about counselling and therapeutic skills and more about support and practical help.

Mental Health Support Workers, with a variety of backgrounds and skills, often provide a service to those with severe mental illnesses, which supports them in daily living in the community, and helps them to remain in the community.

Attempts to define rigidly the boundaries between health and social care and the purchaser and provider functions of managed care can have a negative effect on joint working in mental health services. The need for flexible choice of a worker according to individual skills and needs is paramount. The most recent edition of the *Mental Illness Key Area Handbook* acknowledges,

> "Procedures for nomination or allocation of key workers in community mental health teams continue to cause concern. Priorities need to be established and allocation made in a way that reflects patient need and ensures that differing professional skills are used to the best effect."[21]

Recent guidance on inter-agency working[22] emphasises integration and flexibility in service design and delivery. However, a major issue is the confidentiality of an individual's health records and access to health information. Failure to pass on crucial information was criticised in the Clunis case. The guidance document, *Building Bridges, 1995*, addresses this delicate balance:

- Information given for one purpose may not be disclosed to a third party or used for a different purpose without the consent of the patient.

- The patient should be made aware that, in order for the NHS and local authority social services (or other services such as probation, housing or voluntary agencies) to plan and provide effective care, personal information may need to pass between them.

- Information should be restricted to that in which the recipient has a legitimate interest.

- There may be particular circumstances in which disclosure of information is required by statute or court order or exceptionally, in the absence of consent, can be justified in the public interest.

- It is important to share the right amount of information with those who need to know.

- Decisions on the disclosure of information should be based on the facts, not on supposition or rumour.

RISK AND DANGEROUSNESS

The assessment and management of risk have always been an integral part of practice under the *1983 Mental Health Act* (and earlier legislation), deriving from one of the basic legal grounds for detention: that it may be authorised in the interests of the person's own health or safety or with a view to the protection of other people.

This reflects a recognition that in a minority of cases mental illness may result in violent or dangerous behaviour towards members of the person's household, or acquaintances or professionals involved in the person's care, or towards unknown members of the public. More commonly, it may result in deliberate self harm. A number of highly publicised cases involving the deaths of members of the public or of professionals, have focused attention on the issue of violence by people who are mentally ill, and whether the services delivered to them in the community are sufficient to monitor and manage the risks such people may present. In these cases, mental health difficulties were commonly complicated by drug misuse, homelessness and a history of contact with criminal justice agencies[23,24,25].

Evidence from the USA suggests that there is a slightly increased risk of violent behaviour amongst those with a diagnosis of mental illness. The risk is higher for young men, for those with a diagnosis of schizophrenia, and for those in cases where there is also substance misuse[26]. However, attempts to target or predict particular vulnerable individuals are likely to wrongly identify large numbers of people. In response to the cumulative pressure of a number of enquiries, the present Government has sought to ensure that service targeting takes place and, thereby, the monitoring of vulnerable individuals and their state of mental health. There has been a sustained debate on the issue of compulsory treatment in the community but there are no current proposals to introduce this in the UK.

The Boyd Report[27] into homicides by mentally ill people found that in over half of the cases studied, failure to comply with the treatment plan was a factor in the violent episode. Supervision registers and supervised discharge are both measures designed to provide a framework for supporting and monitoring such individuals. Both of these provisions target particular groups of mentally ill people, including those seen to be at risk of exhibiting violence. One of the aims of both supervision registers and supervised discharge is to ensure compliance with the treatment plan.

The preoccupation with risk and dangerousness, which is a feature of current mental health policy, concentrates attention and resources on the small minority of mentally ill people who present such risks. For professionals working in the community this may mean working assertively with those who are difficult to engage: the evidence is that they are more likely to be younger males, with severe mental illness possibly compounded by drug or alcohol misuse[28]. Non-compliance with medication is likely to be a factor. Community professionals need to be aware of the needs of this challenging clientele, who may now constitute a larger proportion of caseloads.

References

1 Department of Health (1989) *The Care of Children. Principles and Practices in Regulations and Guidance.* Page 8: London: HMSO.

2 Twigg J. and Atkin K.(1994) *Carers Perceived: Policy and Practice in informal Care.* Buckingham: Open University Press.

3 Audit Commission (1994) *Finding a Place: A Review of Mental Health Services for Adults.* London: HMSO.

4 Leff J., Thornicroft G., Coxhead N. and Crawford C. (1994) 'The TAPS Project. 22: A five-year follow-up of long-stay psychiatric patients discharged to the community.' *British Journal of Psychiatry*, 165, (Supplement 25) 13-17.

5 NHS Executive (1996) Circular LASSL(96)16\HSG(96)6 *The Spectrum of Care - a summary of comprehensive local services for people with mental health problems. 24-hour nursed beds for people with severe and enduring mental illness. An audit pack for the Care Programme Approach.* London: Department of Health.

6 Brown P. (1985) *The Transfer of Care.* USA: Routledge and Kegan Paul.

7 Department of Health (1994) *The Health of the Nation Key Area Handbook: Mental Illness.* Second Edition. London: HMSO.

8 Department of Health (1995) *Building Bridges: a guide to arrangements for inter-agency working for the care and protection of severely mentally ill people.* London: Department of Health.

9 Audit Commission (1994) op cit.

10 Hatfield B. and Mohamad H. (1996 in press) 'Case management in mental health services: the role of community mental health support teams.' *Health and Social Care in the Community.*

11 Department of Health (1994) op cit.

MODULE 3

12 Paykel E. (1991) 'Depression in Women'. *British Journal of Psychiatry*, 158, (suppl.10), 22-29.

13 Mirowsky J. and Ross C.E. (1992) 'Age and Depression'. *Journal of Health and Social Behaviour*, 33,187-205.

14 Defeat Depression Campaign (1993) *Defeat Depression: Management Guidelines*. London: Department of Health.

15 Department of Health (1991) *The Patients Charter*. London: HMSO.

16 Department of Health (1995) *Building Bridges: A guide to arrangements for inter-agency working for the care and protection of severely mentally ill people. Health of the Nation*. London: HMSO.

17 NHS Executive (1994) Circular HSG(94)27. *Guidance on the discharge of mentally disordered people and their continuing care in the community*. London; Department of Health.

18 Ritchie J.H., Dick D. and Lingham R. (1994) *The Report of the Inquiry into the Care and Treatment of Christopher Clunis*. London: HMSO.

19 The Woodley Team *Report (1995) Report of the Independent Review Panel to East London and the City Health Authority and Newham Council, following a homicide in July 1994 by a person suffering with a severe mental illness*. London, East London & City HA.

20 Department of Health (1995) Circular HSG(95)8/LAC(95)5. *NHS Responsibilities for meeting Continuing Health Care Needs*. London: Department of Health.

21 Department of Health (1994) op cit.

22 Department of Health (1995) op cit.

23 Ritchie et al (1994) op cit.

24 The Woodley Team Report (1995) op cit.

25 Heginbotham C. (1994) *The Report of the Independent Panel of Inquiry examining the case of Michael Buchanan*. North West London Mental Health NHS Trust.

26 Swanson J.(1994) 'Mental disorder, substance abuse and community violence: an epidemiological approach' in Monahan J. and Steadman H. *Violence and Mental Disorder: Developments in Risk Assessment*. Chicago: University of Chicago Press.

27 Boyd W.D. (1994) *Confidential Inquiry into Homicides and Suicides by Mentally Ill people. A Preliminary Report on Homicide*. London: Steering Committee of the Confidential Inquiry into Homicides and Suicides by Mentally Ill People.

28 Monahan J. and Steadman H.(1994) *Violence and Mental Disorder: Developments in Risk Assessment*. Chicago: University of Chicago Press.

Key Documents

Caring for People. 1989. London: Department of Health.

Working for Patients. 1989. London: Department of Health.

National Health Service and Community Care Act. 1990. London: HMSO.

Specific Grant for the Development of Social Care Services for People with a Mental Illness Circular HC(90)24/LAC(90)10. 1990. London: Department of Health.

The Care Programme Approach for People with a Mental Illness Referred to the Specialist Psychiatric Services Circular HC(90)23/LASSL(90)11. 1990. London: Department of Health.

Introduction of Supervision Registers for Mentally Ill People from 1 April 1994. 1994. Circular HSG(95)5. London: Department of Health.

The Health of the Nation. 1992. London: Department of Health.

The Mental Health Act, 1983. London: HMSO.

The Mental Health (Patients in the Community) Act 1995.
London: HMSO.

Carers (Recognition and Services) Act, 1995.
London: HMSO.

The Children Act, 1989. London: HMSO.

*Review of Health and Social Services for mentally disordered
offenders and others requiring similar services (Reed
Report).* 1992. London: Department of Health and Home
Office.

Mentally disordered offenders: Inter-agency working. 1995.
Circular 12/95. London: Home Office.

*NHS Responsibilities for meeting continuing health care
needs.* 1995. Circular HSG(95)8/LAC(95)5. London:
Department of Health.

*The Spectrum of Care - a summary of comprehensive local
services for people with mental health problems. 24-hour
nursed beds for people with severe and enduring mental
illness. An Audit Pack for the Care Programme Approach.*
Circular LASSL(96)\HSG(96)6. 1996. London: Department of
Health.

• •

This module - "Legislation and Guidance" - is one of 7 modules in "Learning Materials on Mental Health - an Introduction".
The other modules include:

Module 1 - "Recognition of Mental Health Problems"
Module 2 - "Intervention and Management"
Module 4 - "Special Client Groups"
Module 5 - "Special Issues"
Module 6 - "Users, Carers and Children of Parents with Mental Health Problems"
Module 7 - "Sample Training Exercises"

A sister set of materials is also available for professionals involved in assessing risk - " Learning Materials on Mental Health
Risk Assessment"

module 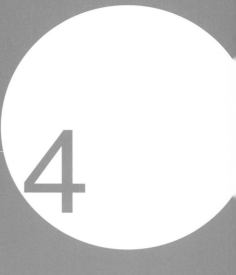 4

SPECIAL CLIENT GROUPS

AIMS & OBJECTIVES

After you have worked through this module you should be better able to:

- Discuss the impact which increased life expectancy will have on the mental health services.
- Identify forms of intervention available for young people with mental health problems.
- Discuss gender differences in mental health and their implications for service.
- Outline the relationships between mental illness and learning disability.
- Evaluate whether members of ethnic minority groups receive fair and appropriate mental health services in the UK.

OLDER PEOPLE WITH MENTAL HEALTH PROBLEMS

As we age, the way we feel about ourselves, and the way other people view us, tends to be affected by loss of friends and family, health and overall status. Older people tend to be undervalued by society and can sometimes be seen as a "nuisance", a "drain" on resources or, simply, "just old". Although those who are seen by services are disabled or experience psychiatric disorders, most older people do not use services and remain active. A range of events do, however, diminish the coping resources of older people.

Examples of events common as we get older include:

- Physical illness, often more than one, affecting different parts of the body. We know how we feel if we have a cold or indigestion or a sore knee, but many older people have all these symptoms all the time or don't have typical symptoms. The pressure of multiple symptoms in vulnerable people whose resistence is lower can have very marked effects.

- Bereavement becomes more likely as we get older. Obviously, the death of a partner is the most painful of all experiences, but the death of close friends, former work colleagues or pets can be equally as painful.

- Loss of status can be problematic: one day you are working, and enjoying the benefits of status and money, then you retire losing status, the money that goes with it and the sense of regular purpose provided by work.

- Loss of normal routine is familiar to many people through, say, a holiday, when you tend to forget what day it is and the lack of a structured day can be disorientating.

The symptoms of the major mental illnesses affecting older people are similar to those experienced by younger people, but there are important differences. Certain mental health problems are commoner in older people.

Dementia is a common condition affecting about 5-10% of people over 65 at any one time and there are about 1% of new cases every year. Dementia rises sharply with age increasing to affect around 25-30% of those over 80 years old. The commonest cause of dementia is Alzheimer's disease, with stroke disease second. Other causes include Lewy body disease and frontal lobe dementia. Other illnesses which can give rise to dementia include Huntington's Chorea, Parkinson's disease and AIDS. (Dementia is discussed in more detail in Module 1).

Depression affects about 5% of older patients, but up to 15% have depressive symptoms which are not severe enough to merit a diagnosis of a clinical depression[1]. Levels of depression can be extremely high amongst patients in wards caring for older people, with up to 50% experiencing some symptoms of a mood disorder. This is also true for residential and nursing home residents. The symptoms of depression in older people are very similar to those in younger patients, with the exception that complaints of physical illness (hypochondriasis) are more common. Often, older clients do not complain of depressive symptoms, but changes in behaviour, such as irritability are prominent. Providing support at periods of loss or change is important. (Depression is discussed in detail in Module 1).

Probably the most common illness in older people is that of **delirium**[2]. A range of physical illnesses in older people, particularly infections, can give rise to delirium. So too can an adverse drug reaction. Delirium is not a mental illness but represents a psychological disturbance caused by a physical illness. An older person who is already known to experience dementia, whose confusion suddenly worsens is most likely to be also suffering from a physical illness which is manifesting itself in the acute confusion. The main indication of delirium is a sudden onset of confusion. There may be problems with attention and concentration, usually causing difficulty in conversation, the person could begin to hallucinate and his or her speech could become rambling.

The condition probably fluctuates over time. Less obvious and dramatic delirium can result from vitamin or hormonal deficiencies and malnutrition.

Paranoid illnesses, often known as **paraphrenia**, can occur at any age. In older people, however, there is sometimes a consistent pattern - patients are usually older women, who often live on their own, have usually never married and seldom have children. They are physically well, although very often have longstanding deafness[3]. Older people with paraphrenia may function well in daily life, but if delusions begin to cause distress or interfere with their functioning, treatment would be indicated.

Other conditions which can cause difficulties in older people include:

- **Anxiety,** which is often not recognised but can sometimes be a sign of an underlying physical illness. Anyone with these symptoms in old age should have a thorough physical examination. Anxiety in older people can indicate an underlying depression.

- **Alcoholism,** which can often be only apparent through circumstantial evidence - and suggestions of drinking too much may often be strenuously denied. Clearly, too much alcohol can complicate any of the illnesses mentioned above. Alcohol dependence can also give rise to secondary health problems such as malnutrition, incontinence and falls. The physical effects of alcohol also increase with age.

- **Physical illness** is often associated with psychiatric symptoms, for example, depression or confusion.

ASSESSMENT

Situations such as those outlined above would normally be catered for in the process of "complex" assessments undertaken under *The NHS and Community Care Act, 1990*. The precise form of "complex" assessment will, of course, differ between local authorities. These assessments are significant in that they focus upon major issues of whether or not a person remains in his or her own home, management of risk, rights and of balancing security against a desire for independence in the face of declining capacity.

RESIDENTIAL AND DAY-CARE ENVIRONMENTS

It is often beneficial to provide older people with mental health difficulties with periods of time out of the home, either for their care and stimulation or to give carers a break. Day care or short-term residential care can enable family carers to "carry on" where, otherwise, permanent residential care may become necessary. Decisions about appropriate care for an older person with dementia need to take into account that a change of environment can lead to further disorientation.

The quality of these care environments is important to the older person, who is entitled to as much privacy and dignity as possible, and should always be treated with respect. As part of a personalised service, attention to detail such as care of clothing and dealing with problems such as incontinence are important. The care setting should offer the right balance between routine and flexibility, and between stimulation and periods of quiet. A regular relationship with a key worker for each person is also important.

CARE SERVICES AT HOME

An individual's needs may be best met by services at home. For some older people, practical help such as shopping or cooking are the most useful service. For others, help with personal tasks, such as getting up, getting dressed, washing and bathing is most needed. These tasks need to be carried out with sensitivity, and respect for people and their homes. Where the older person is highly vulnerable it is important that the provision of all the required services, and the input of carers are organised into an overall plan, designed to reduce and meet potential needs. Such coordinated care is one of the objectives of "intensive" care management. In order to "map" the contribution of services it can be helpful to prepare a timetable of days of the week and key times so as to identify the periods of solitude and maximum risk[4].

For example

	Getting up	Morning	Lunch	Afternoon	Evening	Retiring
Mon						
Tues						
Wed						
Thurs						

CARERS' NEEDS

Carers' needs are interconnected with the difficulties of the older person with a mental health problem. It is therefore important to understand:

- the specific problems of the older person (behaviour, level of functioning),

- the coping attributes of the carer (age, physical frailty and resilience),

- the relationship between carer and "cared for" (both now and in the past), since changes in behaviour and personality may dramatically alter the balance of the relationship,

- the burdens and stresses on the carer (such as loss of social life or work), and

- the impact upon the carer's emotional or psychological well-being.

If there is a regular family carer, services should be geared to giving them support and periods of relief. Sometimes, there may well be conflicts of interest between the carer and the older person. A carer may need a break, but the older person may not want to attend day-care or go into a residential setting. These situations need careful handling. The quality of the alternative care environment may have to be taken into account, along with the likely effects of placement upon both carer and "cared for".

THE RELATIONSHIP BETWEEN THE CARER AND THE OLDER PERSON

If the carer is a member of the family, the quality and history of his or her relationship with the older person will have a bearing on the situation. If the normal relationship has been harmonious, then the care is likely to be given willingly and with affection. If there has been conflict and stress, the dependency may be difficult to accept, and the carer may seem angry or rejecting. Occasionally, the abuse of an older person may be an issue. These situations need skilled assessment and intervention.

• •

DILEMMA

Mr Yates is a 78-year-old man who has had dementia for two years and his memory has consequently deteriorated. He has always been in control of money, has never let his wife deal with their financial affairs and has kept her chronically short of money. Now, with her son's help, she wants to take over the financial affairs and has asked her husband to sign the appropriate forms. He has refused.

What issues might be considered in this situation?

The first thing to do is to make sure you know why everyone has taken their particular position. The understandable reluctance of Mr Yates to give up his role must be acknowledged, as must Mrs Yates' wish to grasp the opportunity at last to have some control of the finances. Such undercurrents usually show themselves as practical problems and families invariably emphasise them.

The important thing is to be objective - the decision is whether Mr Yates can understand what is going on, quite apart from what he decides to do. Anyone can be asked to be an independent witness to the procedure. Power of Attorney was an old piece of legislation which allowed someone to give another person the right to administer his or her affairs, but became void when the person became incapable of making decisions, exactly the time it was needed. Enduring Power of Attorney (EPA) is the modern equivalent. When people cease to be able to understand and make judgements about their affairs, the EPA should be registered with the court of protection so that it can continue. The person has to be capable of understanding that he or she is empowering someone to act for them, if it becomes necessary, at the time the Power of Attorney is signed, so once dementia is established it is too late for Power of Attorney to be given.

In this situation an application needs to be made to the Court of Protection, which makes a decision and then appoints an administrator. This is usually the nearest relative, but may sometimes be local social services and may be a solicitor. These orders are only for financial matters and cannot be used to force a person into a particular type of care.

In certain cases the guardianship provision of *The Mental Health Act, 1983*, has been used. However, in this circumstance it would be appropriate to look beyond the immediate issue of finance for this family since this may be the visible tip of an iceburg of problems. Consider also:

- How they are coping with the changes of role which are necessary and what other pressures are affecting them?

- Who does what in the care of Mr Yates?

- To what extent do they understand what is happening and what understanding does Mr. Yates have of the changes occuring?

- What need does the main carer, Mrs Yates have?

- Does she need some respite from care and from the likely physical demands as well as the daily supervision of her husband?

- Are there areas where appropriate provision of services could prevent pressure and exhaustion building up; leading to his placement in a nursing home or hospital?

What other issues might you consider?

• •

References

1   Katona C. (1994) *Depression in old age*. Chichester: John Wiley.

2   Byrne J. (1994) *Confusional states in older people*. London: Edward Arnold.

3   Pitt B. (1982) *Psychogeriatrics*. Edinburgh: Churchill Livingstone

4 Challis D., Chernum R., Charleman J., Luckett R. and Traske K. (1990) *Care Management in Social and Health Care*. PSSRU. Canterbury: University of Kent.

Further Reading

Bond J., Coleman P. and Peace S. (1994) *Aging in Society - an Introduction to Social Gerontology*. (Second edition.) London: Sage Publication.

Burns A. and Levy R. (1994) *Dementia*. London: Chapman and Hall Medical.

Letts P. (1990) *Managing Other People's Money*. England: Age Concern.

Norman A. (1980) *Rights and Risks*. London: National Corporation for the Care of Old People (now Centre for Policy on Aging).

Norman A. (1985) *Triple Jeopardy - Growing Old in a Second Homeland*. London: Centre for Policy on Aging.

Stephenson O. (1989). *Age and Vulnerability* - Age Concern Handbook. London: Edward Arnold for Hodder and Stoughton Ltd.

YOUNG PEOPLE WITH MENTAL HEALTH PROBLEMS

PREVALENCE

Mental health problems are relatively common in young people, although severe mental illness is rare. Rather than think in terms of illness and disease, therefore, it is perhaps more helpful to think of problems and disorders. A problem has been defined as "a disturbance of function in one area of relationships, mood, behaviour or development, of sufficient severity to require professional assistance"[1]. Examples include bed wetting, sleep disturbance, tantrums or irrational fear of one particular thing, occurring at a stage of development when they would not be expected. Educational difficulty or abdominal pain with no physical cause are other examples. A disorder, then, can be thought of as "either a severe problem (commonly persistent) or the co-occurrence of a number of problems"[2].

Estimates vary as to what proportion of children experience such difficulties, but 10-20% has recently been suggested[3]. Higher rates are known to occur among children in the inner cities compared to rural areas. Many more are likely to be affected than ask for help, since, unlike adults, children are dependent on their carers for recognising symptoms and seeking advice. Children with behavioural problems are probably referred more frequently than those with emotional difficulties, which cause less trouble to other people. The accessibility of local services is also an important consideration.

A recent large-scale American study[4], found that the. proportion of children with significant problems is similar across different age groups, but the type of disorder varies with sex and age. Boys up to 16 showed far more behavioural disorders than girls, and girls over 12 more anxiety and depressive disorders than boys. Though some very disabling conditions, for example, autism, become apparent in the early years, it is mainly in adolescence that adult-type mental illnesses (schizophrenia and major depressive disorders) begin to be seen. Eating disorders, deliberate self-harm and substance abuse are also less common before puberty.

CAUSES

Although it sometimes seems obvious why a particular child develops a mental health problem, it is often harder to explain why another, in similar circumstances, remains apparently unaffected. Almost invariably, the cause is due to many factors. For example, an already vulnerable child is likely to develop psychological difficulties in an especially stressful situation. It is useful, therefore, to think of interacting risk factors which are related to the child, the family or the environment, and may well have a different impact according to age.

Risk factors specific to the individual child include:

* genetic inheritance (which seems to predispose certain individuals to some disorders);

* temperament;

* chronic or severe physical illness or injury; and

* difficulties with learning and communication.

All of them may affect self-esteem and interpersonal relationships. Risk factors associated with the family are particularly significant. Lack of an early attachment to a consistent, loving care-giver has been linked with subsequent psychiatric conditions[5]. These ideas have since been reappraised to some extent[6], but the importance of secure attachment is still generally acknowledged.

Young people growing up need a family where there is recognition of their developmental needs, an accepting attitude and clear, consistent discipline. Abuse, emotional, physical or sexual, is strongly linked to psychiatric disorders. Problems associated with the parents themselves also create risk. For example, family breakdown, marital discord, mental illness and criminality are all more frequent in the backgrounds of children with mental health difficulties.

Environmental risk includes both the circumstances of everyday living, such as socio-economic disadvantage and discrimination, and also single critical life events.

On the other hand, positive characteristics in the young person, such as self-esteem, sociability and a sense of autonomy, a warm, cohesive family and adequate social support, including perhaps a positive school experience, can provide protection[7].

CLASSIFICATION

Like adult mental disorders, those of childhood have been medically classified to facilitate communication and research. In practice, however, it is often difficult to categorise them specifically. Indeed, people often experience more than one condition, for example, mixed emotional and conduct disorder. Two fairly similar diagnostic systems are used, the American DSM-IV and the World Health Organisation ICD-10, both are updated from time to time in the light of current thinking. Here is a simplified summary:

- **Emotional disorders** - anxiety, phobias, mild depression, obsessive-compulsive disorder.

- **Conduct Disorders** - non-compliant oppositional behaviour, stealing, fire-setting, aggression, substance abuse.

- **Hyperactive Disorders** - attention deficit hyperactive disorder.

- **Developmental Disorders** - either specific, for example, in speech and language, or pervasive, for example, autism.

- **Eating Disorders** - anorexia nervosa, bulimia.

- **Psychotic Disorders** - schizophrenia, major depression, mania.

- **Somatic Disorders** - chronic fatigue syndrome.

Apparently similar behaviour, such as refusing to go to school or self-harm, may express different underlying problems.

Example of a young person with a conduct disorder

Tom is a 12-year-old boy, who is disruptive in lessons, aggressive in the playground and plays truant some days. At home he fights constantly with his siblings, is disobedient, cheeky to his divorced mother and steals money for cigarettes. He has been admitted to hospital following a cocktail of tablets and alcohol which he took with friends for a dare.

Example of young person with an emotional disorder

Olivia is a 13-year-old girl, who has always been rather anxious and fearful . At school she is a perfectionist and does well academically, but has found the move to high school very stressful, feels lonely and often misses days with headaches and unexplained sickness. After an argument with her mother about this, she takes an overdose of paracetamol in her bedroom.

CONTINUITY INTO ADULT LIFE

Many young people who experience mental health problems will outgrow them. There is some correlation between psychological difficulty in childhood and adulthood, but it is not easy to predict on an individual level. Some conditions, however, are known to have a better prognosis. With increasing maturity, developmental delays tend to be minimised and hyperactivity may lessen, though other symptoms may remain and are associated with anti-social behaviour as an adult. Emotional disorders often improve, although obsessional-compulsive disorders are likely to persist. It has been suggested[8] that depression in childhood may be less transitory than was previously thought and tends to recur episodically in adulthood. The outcome for conduct disorders is less good; in about a third of cases they persist into adult life, and may then be associated with not only anti-social, but also depressive, disorders. The former are more common in men and the latter in women[9].

INTERVENTION

Because many factors cause most childhood mental disorders, intervention is usually a complex task. However, it needs to be undertaken to try to minimise the distress of the young person and the effects on those closely associated with him or her. Shortening the duration of a mental health problem can also reduce the risk of secondary handicap. For example, time away from school, either because of anxiety or exclusion for poor behaviour, may lead to educational and subsequent socio-economic disadvantage. Psychiatric treatment alone is rarely adequate. Other services are likely to have a role and need to work together, including primary health care, social services, education and possibly juvenile justice.

Activity

Talk to a local teacher and ask how adolescents with emotional or behavioural disorders are dealt with in mainstream school.

Recent government publications have recommended that treatment should be provided in four tiers, the first being "Primary or Direct Contact Services"[10, 11, 12]. The other three tiers include:

- **Tier 2** - Interventions offered by the individual staff of specialist child and adolescent mental health services

- **Tier 3** - Services offered by multi-disciplinary teams of staff from specialist child and adolescent mental health services

- **Tier 4** - Very specialised interventions and care

Specialist child and adolescent mental health services, which offer treatment for more severe and complex disorders, have been criticised as patchy at present[13]. Names of treatment centres vary, but often they are called Child and/or Family Guidance Clinics or Child and Adolescent Psychiatry Departments in hospitals. Day patient or inpatient facilities may sometimes be available for more intensive assessment or treatment. The professional team is likely to include psychiatrists, clinical or educational psychologists, nurses, possibly social workers and various therapists, such as psychotherapists, occupational, play and, occasionally, art or music therapists.

The type of treatment offered will depend on what current research suggests is likely to be effective, but also on the professionals involved and the availability of resources.

Individual, family or group interventions are all used. Most treatments will be largely based on talking with parents and children, though drugs may be prescribed for a limited number of conditions. Partly because of economic constraints, interventions tend to be short-term and focused, although occasionally longer-term regular psychodynamic work may be undertaken with a child.

Behavioural programmes based on learning theory are often used for conduct problems and, currently, cognitive behavioural therapy, which takes into account individual thoughts and feelings, is being developed for use with depressed adolescents.

Many departments offer family therapy and working with parents is generally an important part of treatment. Whichever method is chosen, it is necessary that the circumstances of the young person's life are sufficiently supportive to enable it to succeed. Any behavioural programme, for instance, needs to be consistently administered by the child's carers. Trying to treat unwilling recipients is not usually productive, but life-threatening situations may occur, for example, in cases of self harm or starvation, when such action may be considered justifiable. The compulsory provisions of *The Mental Health Act, 1983*, apply to all age groups.

● ●

DILEMMA

Michael is a fifteen year old whose family you have recently become involved with. He lives at home with his mother, stepfather and three stepbrothers. During his adolescence Michael has frequently been in trouble with the police for stealing and he regularly truants from school. Recently he has become particularly aggressive towards his mother and has also threatened to harm himself. Michael's mother tried to take him to visit his GP today but he has refused to go. You are a child care social worker and arrive in the middle of a heated dispute about this. His mother informs you that Michael has been "acting strangely" refusing to get out of bed and expressing ideas that people are out to get him.

What might you consider?

- Check the information. (If Michael will cooperate, try to interview him separately - unless you feel there is a risk of Michael being violent towards you)

- Is this normal adolescent behaviour? What is happening with his family, school, peers.

- Is there a possibility of substance abuse?

- Is Michael a risk to himself or others? How serious is the threat of self harm?

- Is Michael in need of urgent medical/psychiatric assessment?

- If so, can the GP visit?

- If not, do you need to contact an Approved Social Worker for a Mental Health Act assessment?

- If the situation seems less urgent, should you involve Child Psychiatry and how do you do this?

What other issues might you consider?

● ●

IMPLICATIONS FOR SOCIAL SERVICES

Social services are probably in the best position of all agencies to reduce some of the risk factors associated with child mental health problems, particularly those linked with the family and socio-economic disadvantage. It is, therefore, crucial that they are involved in joint planning with health and education in providing an effective service[14]. The boundaries between the services cannot be drawn distinctly.

For people working within social services, especially those involved with adult mental health and children and families, issues related to child mental health perhaps occur more frequently than is generally recognised. Often, however, they may be only too apparent and call for difficult judgements to be made.

References

1   Wallace, S.A., Crown, J.M., Cox, A.D., and Berger, M., (1995) *Epidemiologically Based Needs Assessment: Child and Adolescent Mental Health.* London: DOH.

2   Wallace, S.A. et al. Ibid.

3   Social Services Inspectorate (1995) *A Handbook on Child and Adolescent Mental Health.* London: HMSO.

4   Cohen, P., Cohen, J.,Kasen, S., Velez, C.N., Hartmark, C., Johnson, J., Rojas,M., Brook, J., and Streuning, E.L., An epidemiological study of disorders in late childhood and adolescence - 1. Age and gender-specific prevalence. *Journal of Child Psychology and Psychiatry*, 34, 851-867.

5   Bowlby, J. (1969). *Attachment and Loss: Vol.1: Attachment.* London: Hogarth Press.

6   Rutter, M., (1972) *Maternal Deprivation Reassessed.* Harmonsdsworth: Penguin.

7   Rutter, M., (1989) Pathways from Childhood to adult life. *Journal of Child Psychology and Psychiatry*, 30, 23-51.

8   Harrington, R ., *Depressive Disorder in Childhood and Adolescence.* Chichester: John Wiley.

9   Quinton,D., Rutter, M., and Gulliver, L., (1990). *Continuities in psychiatric disorders from childhood to adulthood in the children of psychiatric patients.* In L.N. Robins and M. Rutter (ed.) *Straight and devious pathways from childhood to adulthood.* Cambridge: Cambridge University Press.

10 Social Services Inspectorate (1995) op cit.

11 Health Advisory Service (1995) *Together We Stand.* London: HMSO.

12 Department of Health. *A Handbook on Child and Adolescent Mental Health. The Health of the Nation.* London: SSI of the Department of Health, joint publication with the Department for Education.

13 Health Advisory Service (1995) op cit.

14 Health Advisory Service (1995) op cit.

Further Reading

Barker, P.,(1995) *Basic Child Psychiatry* (sixth edition).
Oxford: Blackwell.

Children's Law Centre (1994) *Young People, Mental Health
and the Law - A Handbook for Parents and Advisers.*
Colchester: Essex University.

WOMEN AND MENTAL HEALTH

INTRODUCTION

In the early 1970s different rates of mental health difficulty between men and women began to be discussed in relation to the different social role expectations of the sexes. An influential paper identified that the rates of referral for psychiatric help were markedly different between the sexes for married men and women, but that differences were less consistently reported for the single or the separated and divorced[1]. Married women emerged as particularly prone to mental health problems, when compared with married men. The authors suggested that this may be due to the nature of the married woman's social role; this was described as "frustrating", a position of "low prestige" and "unstructured and invisible". Women were identified as being disadvantaged in the workplace, and when women did go out to work, they were overburdened because of their domestic tasks.

Since the 1970s there have been substantial changes in family structures, which render comparisons between "married" and "not married" as too simple. Many adults spend time in intimate partner relationships which may be neither "marriages" nor permanent. Children are often looked after in complex family arrangements which may include step-parents and step-siblings or other household relationships.

Changes which may have implications for the mental health of women are the substantial increase in lone parenthood since the 1970s, and the increase in the proportion of mothers of young children in the workforce.

COMMON MENTAL HEALTH PROBLEMS

The common mental health difficulties of depression and anxiety are consistently identified more often in women[2]. A range of reasons for this has been suggested. The first of these is that women are more likely to seek help for their distress. The expression of distress is seen to be more socially acceptable in women. Support for this explanation comes from a range of studies showing women's greater willingness to consult their doctor[3]. The over-representation of men in suicides and in alcohol misuse also suggests a pattern of behaviours which may reflect avoidance of seeking help. However, community surveys, involving those who have not sought specific help, also show a marked excess of women with common mental health difficulties.

A substantial amount of investigation has focused upon the experience of depression in women. Biological explanations have been one avenue of exploration. Hormonal changes following childbirth appear to play a part in post-natal depression, although relationship factors also contribute[4,5]. However, the evidence suggests that the contribution of female biology to the development of depression is limited, and that other factors are more significant.

Further research has followed the directions set in the early 1970s, in relation to the links between the mental health of women and their social role. Since the 1970s, there have been marked social changes affecting the life situations of many women. The relationship between some of these specific factors and the mental health of women are discussed below.

Partners and children

The findings of a range of studies indicate that women with young children are at particular risk of developing depression[6,7]. Many studies have found an increased rate of minor mental health problems in women with young children, but not men - single men emerge as more at risk. Brown and Harris identified in 1978 that about a quarter of working-class women with young children in their sample experienced depression following a serious life event[8]. However, this was less likely if women had a confiding relationship with a partner, or if they had paid work outside of the home. These acted as "protective factors".

In modern Western society, women have the primary responsibility for the care and nurture of young children. The evidence is that this role can lead to an increased likelihood of poor mental health for women. Despite this, there has been only limited support offered in social policy measures for women with young children. Public child care, enabling women to work is in very limited supply, whilst measures enabling male parents to contribute more equally to the care of children have implications for the workplace which have been resisted.

Employment

Paid employment outside of the home is generally seen to offer rewards supportive of individual mental health, these include:

- the opportunity for relationships,

- remuneration,

- an enhanced sense of personal competence, and

- a valued social role.

However, for women caring for young children, their employment outside the home has a rather more varied impact. A number of studies have examined the relationship between work and mental health for women with children. For those caring for children under school-age, full-time employment increases the risk of minor mental health problems, but part-time work appears to have a protective effect[9,10]. One study of professional women, working full-time with young children, found that women were more psychologically distressed if they believed they could not rely upon their partners to share the child care[11]. Such studies suggest that women who work full-time and take major responsibility for young children are particularly at risk. Lone mothers face particularly bleak choices; the identification of the "feminization of poverty"[12] in the USA focuses on the increasing proportions of children being reared in poverty by lone mothers. A Canadian study of a group of 356 women found that those reporting anxiety or depression were more likely to be relatively poor and without partners[13].

Women as carers

Numerous surveys have identified that for adults who need care by virtue of illness, disability or frailty in old age, the likelihood is that they will be looked after by a female relative, although a minority of such carers are male[14,15]. Whatever the reason for the need for care, caring is a highly stressful task and the mental health of carers is generally reported to be poor[16,17]. In one study of mothers of children with severe learning disabilities, the mental health of the mothers was found to be poor but that of the fathers did not differ from the general population[18]. In this study gender roles within the families allowed fathers to lead relatively normal working lives, but the opportunities of the mothers were severely restricted. This sort of evidence has led to challenges to the concept of "community care" - which may place greater burdens on carers[19,20].

Commonly, women who have brought up children then become carers of adults in mid-life - both situations of increased mental health vulnerability. Support services for carers often do not provide enough relief from care to enable those caring to have the opportunity for paid work or leisure activities. Studies show that the caring responsibility is not usually shared within families, but tends to fall upon one individual.

The recent *Carers (Recognition and Services) Act, 1995*, requires Local Authorities to take account of the needs of carers, placing the needs of carers on the agenda of care management.

Activity

Think about the people you know - family, friends and colleagues.
- Do the women and men experience different pressures in their lives?
- Are there factors which have a more pronounced impact on the well-being of men?
- Do the pressures on the lives of the women you know reflect those identified in the above account?

SEVERE AND LONG-TERM MENTAL ILLNESS

People with severe mental illnesses (usually the psychotic illnesses) are now looked after in the community where possible, though many will spend short periods of time in hospital. Increased community living has proved to have different implications for men and women. Schizophrenia, the most common of the severe mental illnesses, occurs in men at a younger age and with more disabling symptoms[21,22]. Possibly as a consequence of this, men with schizophrenia are less likely to marry or have children than men in the general population[23].

Women with severe mental illnesses are more likely than men to live in families, or to have a partner or children[24]. Evidence from the USA where the "de-institutionalisation" of people with severe mental illness has progressed rapidly, is that few programmes of support offer the sort of care needed by these women Their parenting skills are likely to be seriously deficient, and the risks of losing their children to the public care system are high.

In community care settings, such as those which offer day care or residential care in groups for those with the more severe mental health difficulties, men often out-number women service users. This may be because women are more likely to retain their family connections; or it may be a product of the later onset and less severe symptoms of schizophrenia which tend to occur in women, reducing the overall need. However, thought needs to be given to the attractiveness of service settings for women where severely disabled men are the predominant users. "Women only" facilities are often a more sensitive alternative for meeting women's needs.

A degree of security can also be provided in "women only" settings for women who have been physically or sexually abused by men in the past. This is particularly an issue for the special hospitals, where many of the women detained have histories of abuse, and the facility also provides services for men, some of whom will be serious sex offenders.

For women looking after young children, there can be major practical difficulties in keeping appointments or using services which fail to take account of the timing of women's child care commitments. Women with mental health difficulties may not be well resourced to create and maintain reciprocal arrangements for child care with other mothers.

POLICY AND PRACTICE IN COMMUNITY CARE

The limited resources for helping people with mental health problems have increasingly become prioritised in favour of those with more severe and enduring difficulties. Further priority within this group is now meant to be given to individuals who present serious risks such as violence or self-harm. This means that workers in the community cannot respond to all mental health need, but have to prioritise certain key groups.

Such priority systems operate to exclude as well as include. Our concern is that the criteria for specialist services may result in the exclusion of greater numbers of women with mental health needs. This is because fewer women will present with severe psychotic illness and high levels of risk, particularly risk of violence. However, more women experience the common mental health problems of, for example, depression. Current government policy is for GPs and the primary care team to address this level of need. It remains to be seen whether a sufficient range of therapeutic support can be developed outside of specialist services. Social work support within care management arrangements is likely to be limited, unless there are high levels of social need.

WOMEN'S MENTAL HEALTH NEEDS

The psycho-social contribution to women's mental health difficulties appears to spring from widely-held beliefs about the social role of women, particularly in relation to family care and the workplace. These will have different significance according to the age and life stage of women. Whilst social role expectations will also affect men detrimentally, the mental health impact is perhaps less widespread.

Approaches to helping women with mental health difficulties have incorporated an understanding of women's changing social roles across the life span[25,26]. Psycho-social issues relevant to a woman in her 30s may be less relevant to a woman in her 60s, when different losses, changes and tasks will present themselves.

These approaches include helping the individual woman gain an understanding of her own life situation, and enhancing self-esteem and self-efficacy. Psycho-social approaches should ideally be an integral part of multi-disciplinary assessment and treatment planning. Their aim will be to enhance the understanding and control of the individual.

Good practices in the provision of mental health services for women have been identified as:

Services which

- promote self-esteem;

- provide care to the woman in her own right;

- provide space to talk through feelings and experiences in a non-threatening atmosphere;

- enable the woman to take control of her own life;

- acknowledge that bad feelings are common to everyone;

- acknowledge the "normality" of mental distress.

Services also need to:

- be accessible, without women having to leave children or have them taken into care;

- provide the opportunity to meet with other women in similar circumstances;

- provide access to sources of practical help as well as to counselling, therapy and drug treatments;

- enable the woman to receive help from a female worker if that is her choice[27].

References

1   Gove W.R. and Tudor J.F.(1973) 'Adult sex roles and mental illness'. *American Journal of Sociology*, 78:4, 812-835.

2   Office of Population Censuses and Surveys (1994) *OPCS surveys of psychiatric morbidity in Great Britain: Bulletin No.1. The prevalence of psychiatric morbidity among adults aged 16-64 living in private households in Great Britain.* London: OPCS.

3   Goldberg D. and Huxley P. (1980) *Mental Illness in the Community: the pathway to psychiatric care.* London: Tavistock.

4   Paykel E.S.(1991) 'Depression in women'. *British Journal of Psychiatry*, 158, (Suppl.10), 22-29.

5   Murray D.,Cox J.L., Chapman G. and Jones P.(1995) 'Childbirth: Life event or start of a long-term difficulty? Further data from the Stoke-on-Trent controlled study of post-natal depression.' *British Journal of Psychiatry*, 166, 595-600.

6   Brown G.W. and Harris T. (1978) *Social Origins of Depression: a study of psychiatric disorders in women.* London: Tavistock.

7   Elliott B.J. and Huppert F.A. (1991) 'In sickness and in health: associations between physical and mental well-being, employment and parental status in a British nationwide sample of married women'. *Psychological Medicine*, 21, 515-524.

8   Brown and Harris (1978) op cit.

9   Elliott and Huppert (1991) op cit.

10   Brown G.W. and Bifulco A.(1990) 'Motherhood, employment and the development of depression: a replication of a finding?' *British Journal of Psychiatry*, 156, 169-179.

11   Ozer E.M.(1995) 'The impact of childcare responsibility and self-efficacy on the psychological health of professional working mothers'. *Psychology of Women Quarterly*, 19, 315-335.

12 Rodgers H.R.(1990) *Poor women, poor families: the economic plight of America's female-headed households.* New York: M.E.Sharpe inc.

13 Walters V.(1993) 'Stress, anxiety and depression: women's accounts of their health problems.' *Science and Medicine*, 36,4, 393-402.

14 Twigg J.(1994) *Carers perceived: policy and practice in informal care.* Buckingham: Open University Press.

15 Levin E., Moriarty J. and Gorbach P.(1994) *Better for the break.* National Institute for Social Work Research Unit. London: HMSO.

16 Twigg J. (1994) op cit.

17 Levin E. et al, (1994) op cit.

18 Wilkin D.(1979) *Caring for the Mentally Handicapped Child.* London: Croom Helm.

19 Brown H. and Smith H.(1989) 'Whose 'ordinary life' is it any way?' *Disability, Handicap and Society*, 4,2, 105-119.

20 Finch J. and Groves D.(1983) *A Labour of Love: women, work and caring.* London: Routledge and Kegan Paul.

21 Castle D.J., Wessely,S. and Murray R.M.(1993) 'Sex and schizophrenia: effects of diagnostic stringency and associations with premorbid varaiables', *British Journal of Psychiatry*, 162, 658-664.

22 Lewis S.(1992) 'Sex and schizophrenia: vive la difference', *British Journal of Psychiatry*, 161, 445-450.

23 Lane A., Byrne M.,Mulvaney F., Kinsella A., Addington J.L., Walsh D., Larkin C. and O'Callaghan E.(1995) 'Reproductive behaviour in schizophrenia relative to other mental disorders: evidence for increased fertility in men despite decreased marital rate', *Acta Psychiatrica Scandinavica*, 91, 222-228.

24 Test M.A., Burke S.S. and Wallisch L.S.(1990) 'Gender differences of young adults with schizophrenic disorders in community care', *Schizophrenia Bulletin*, 16,2, 331-344.

25 Barnes M. and Maple N. (1992) *Women and Mental Health: Challenging the stereotypes.* Birmingham: Venture Press.

26 Scarf M. (1980) *Unfinished Business: pressure points in the lives of women.* USA: Fontana.

27 Good Practices in Mental Health/ European Regional Council World Federation for Mental Health (1994) *Women and Mental Health. An Information Pack of mental Health Services for Women in the United Kingdom.* London: GPMH Publications.

THE PSYCHIATRY OF LEARNING DISABILITY
(MENTAL HANDICAP)

MODULE 4

The American Association on Mental Retardation defines learning disability as "substantial limitations in present functioning. It is characterised by significantly subaverage intellectual functioning, existing concurrently with related limitations in two or more of the following applicable adaptive skill areas: communication, self-care, home living, social skills, community use, self-direction, health and safety, functional academics, leisure and work. Mental retardation manifests before age 18."[1]. In the UK, most people in contact with learning disability services have an IQ of 60-65 or lower. However, people of higher IQ who have additional problems, particularly behaviour problems, may also be in contact with these services.

The psychiatry of learning disability is a relatively new field, so the provision of specialist psychiatric services to this population is still fairly patchy. However, an increasing number of psychiatrists are now being trained specifically in this discipline, and sometimes work as members of the Community Support Team itself. Further new developments include the publishing of training materials and schedules for front-line workers and other staff. These are designed to help raise awareness about the manifestations of mental disorders in this population, and to collect information about mental health in a systematic way, to enable decisions about possible referrals to be made on a more informed basis. These materials are discussed shortly.

There are many factors which suggest that people with learning disability are more at risk for developing mental health problems than the general population. One only needs to reflect on the possibility of genetic abnormalities, birth trauma, parental rejection, institutionalisation, social stigmatisation and lack of friends, to recognise the potential for mental illness to develop. Not surprisingly, evidence from large scale studies of morbidity indicates that people with learning disability have higher rates for psychoses and autism, and a very high rate for challenging behaviour, compared with the general population[2]. There are so many possible influences that it is often very difficult to say if presenting behaviours are the result of an organic condition, a psychiatric disorder, environmental influences or a combination of these. For many years we have known that learning disability and psychiatric disorders frequently coexist, but only recently has the psychiatry of learning disability been given close attention. Researchers and health care professionals are aware that we are not always successful in meeting the mental health needs of these people[3]. The difficulties of detecting and diagnosing psychiatric conditions in this population group is undoubtedly one of the reasons for this situation. Carers may not realize that a problem is due to illness, or that help may be available by consulting a doctor. Doctors may find it difficult to decide whether the problem is an illness, or to make a confident diagnosis.

It is vital that we deal with such issues. Behavioural and psychiatric disorders often determine the level of specialist support someone needs to live independently in the community. The joint contributions of mental illness, problematic behaviour and learning disability produce a group of people whose quality of life will continue to be seriously impaired, unless they are diagnosed and treated effectively.

Activity

- In your area which services are provided for people with both learning disabilities and mental health problems?

- Are the services provided the most suitable for the needs of these people?

PREVALENCE

The most common high-profile conditions of people with learning disabilities are challenging behaviours, particularly aggression and self injury. Severe behaviour problems are the most common reason in the UK for referral to a psychiatrist, accounting for more than half the presentations among long-stay residents and a third of admissions from the community. These behaviour problems are often long term and we cannot predict how long they will last. They often do not fit the established criteria for a diagnosable psychiatric condition and their inclusion or exclusion of problem behaviours has a major influence on apparent prevalence.

There is, therefore, considerable uncertainty about defining mental illness in people with learning disability to estimate prevalence. Despite the uncertainty, evidence from large scale studies suggests that, across the spectrum of mental disorder, the pattern of prevalence is different than it is among people in general. Schizophrenia is reported as being up to 20 times more likely among people in this group than generally[4], whilst affective and neurotic disorders are less likely. (However, this latter finding probably reflects the problems of detecting anxiety and depression in this population, rather than being a genuinely lower prevalence than the general population[5]). Autistic disorders are also very much more prevalent in people with learning disabilities and it can be difficult to distinguish the symptoms of autism from those of psychosis in adults.

Clearly we need to be cautious about current prevalence figures. There is much work to be done in validating diagnostic methods for people with learning disabilities.

PSYCHIATRIC PROBLEMS OF OLDER INDIVIDUALS

Since the turn of the century most industrial countries have seen a marked shift in the age structure of their populations. Obviously, the improvement in the quality of medical care has increased life expectancy. People are now much more likely to survive serious illness in old age than they were 50 years ago. For people with learning disabilities, some of whom tend to be more prone to illness, medical advances have had an even greater impact. The increasing number of older people increases age-related health problems.

Dementia is one of the disorders most obviously associated with the process of ageing and the link with Down's syndrome is now recognised. Evidence suggests that the brains of many (or all) people with Down's syndrome, who are aged 35 or over, show the characteristic changes associated with dementia. At the same time, it is important to bear in mind that the relationship between the behavioural symptoms and brain abnormality is not at all clear. While medical evidence is considered conclusive, clinical symptoms may not be. A person with Down's syndrome is often diagnosed after death as having Alzheimer's disease, even if there have been no observable clinical symptoms. It is most important not to jump to the conclusion that behaviour apparently symptomatic of dementia necessarily indicates the onset of this disease. A variety of conditions, many of them treatable, can mimic the early symptoms of dementia. A full clinical examination, and monitoring for at least six months, are necessary before a firm conclusion can be reached.

Research in Oldham, Lancashire, on people with learning disabilities who were aged over 50 indicated a dementia prevalence rate of around 11% to 12%[6]. Although by this age there were only nine people with learning disabilities out of 105 people, five of these were found to have dementia - an indication of the high risk for these individuals. However, while the link between Alzheimer's disease and Down's syndrome is well recognised, it is often forgotten that, because of their reduced life expectancy, people with Down's syndrome represent a fairly small proportion of the over-50s. There are probably more people with dementia and learning disabilities who do not have Down's syndrome, than those who do. Many of the people with a firm diagnosis of dementia deteriorated in caring for themselves and in their community skills. This, coupled with their generally poor health, suggests that their needs call for a major use of social service resources.

THE PATHWAY TO CARE

In considering their mental health needs it is important to consider the extent to which psychiatric conditions are socially defined. Some social situations seem able to contain or deal with the psychiatric symptoms. Others, produce or exacerbate them. Interaction between the individual and his or her family may be a major source of support, enabling the effects of, for instance, depression to be minimised. Also possible is that the family is a major source of conflict, actually raising the severity of the condition, and certainly making it more possible that the individual comes to the attention of medical services. Whether or not someone seeks professional help depends largely on these effects. For most people, it is the GP who is the most important filter on the path to psychiatric help. The first visit to the doctor usually occurs when it becomes clear to others that there has been some change in the person's behaviour or ability to cope. The onset of a mental health problem is often heralded by being unable to hold down a job or go on successfully as a parent and spouse. The GP decides if the patient has significant mental illness, and can be treated by the doctor or referred to a psychiatrist.

Many people with learning disabilities, however, have far fewer formal "roles". They tend not to be parents or spouses. They often have less demanding jobs. As a result, there may not be any dramatic, outward signs of significant depression or anxiety, although distress to the individual may be considerable. Without specialist knowledge, the symptoms may be seen as part of the learning disability and referral to the GP for further psychiatric evaluation may not be made.

So, the pathway to psychiatric care involves at least two steps. Firstly, people who know the person have to notice a significant change in behaviour. Secondly, the person has come to the attention of a medical practitioner. Because of the way this pathway works, certain conditions are more likely to be detected than others. Alcohol abuse or schizophrenia are more noticeable than depression or anxiety, because they often result in "high profile" behaviour which is easily noticed and often causes a nuisance to others. As a result, only a fraction of the people with mental health problems in the community come to the attention of psychiatric services. The problem of detecting mental illness among people with learning disabilities is even more difficult. Research so far shows that many of them remain undetected and so have little prospect of being treated properly. This shows how important it is to focus, not just on developing psychiatric techniques, but on improving the pathway of appropriate treatment for these people.

IMPROVING DETECTION OF MENTAL HEALTH PROBLEMS

The difficulties of detecting and diagnosing psychiatric conditions in this population group is undoubtedly one of the reasons why there is such a high level of unmet psychiatric need in people with learning disability. Ensuring that people with learning disability get appropriate help for their mental health problems is not just a job for psychiatrists. Health and social service staff have an essential role in ensuring that people who have psychiatric problems are identified and referred for comprehensive assessment. This, in turn, implies that they need access to information about the manifestation of mental illnesses in people with learning disability, the tools to provide a systematic framework with which this information can be collected, and guidance on who should be referred for further psychiatric assessment. Attention is drawn to a recent collaboration between the Hester Adrian Research Centre and UDMS Guy's and St. Thomas's Hospital, to provide a multi-level approach to the detection and diagnosis of mental disorders. *Mental Health and Learning Disabilities* is a training pack for front-line staff and other health professionals[7]. This pack is modular in structure, and is hence flexible for use with staff who are new to the field as well as those who already have some knowledge.

The pack also includes two new schedules to enable staff to collect systematic information on the mental health of the people for whom they care, and to make informed decisions on whom to refer for further psychiatric assessment. The *PAS-ADD Checklist* is a short schedule couched in everyday language, designed for use primarily by care staff and families - the people who have the most immediate perception of changes in the behaviour of the individuals for whom they care. The Checklist aims to help staff and carers decide whether further assessment of an individual's mental health may be helpful. It can be used to screen whole groups of individuals, or as part of a regular monitoring of people who are considered to be at risk of mental illness. The *Mini-PAS-ADD* is a more detailed questionnaire, designed to provide a fuller assessment of current mental health. It is targeted primarily at clinical psychologists, community nurses, social workers and other professionals working with adults who have a learning disability, and aims to give a more informed basis for decisions about possible referral for further psychiatric assessment.

ASSESSMENT AND TREATMENT

It is crucial for the effective treatment of mental disorders that assessment is as comprehensive as possible. Diagnostic methods for people with learning disabilities and mental illness are no different fundamentally from those used with other people. However, the poor verbal ability of many of them is clearly an obstacle to psychiatric interviewing. They are likely to find it difficult to express their emotions verbally, as a result of which many studies have relied on third-party reports for information on which to make a diagnosis. Information from key people is vital to the detection and assessment of their condition, but confidence in a diagnosis based solely on third party reports cannot be high. The rules of good interviewing in this context are not basically different from those generally followed. But there are two particularly important points to bear in mind. Firstly, people with learning disabilities are more likely to say what they believe the interviewer wants to hear. Secondly, they often have a relatively short attention span. In addition, a wide variety of speech and hearing problems can make the client difficult to understand. The interviewer should be particularly aware of the more subtle problems which can lead to misunderstanding, notably, poor grammar and abnormal intonation. Clinical interviewing of people with learning disabilities is a skill which demands in-depth training and sensitivity to their problems, whether or not they have a mental health problem.

In people who have little or no language, changes in behaviour can be the first sign of a developing mental disorder. Detailed information from the client and other people is essential. The clinical picture can sometimes be very complicated, especially if a psychiatric disorder is associated with, or concurrent with, an existing challenging behaviour. Evaluating the contribution of biological, psychological, social, family and environmental factors to the observed signs and symptoms may call for repeated assessments, and, in some cases, the use of direct observation. Treatment may include the full range of psychological and pharmacological interventions, as well as the treatment of physical illness and/or sensory impairments.

References

1   American Association on Mental Retardation (AAMR), (1992). *Mental Retardation: Definition, Classification and Systems of Supports*. Washington: AAMR.

2   Holland, A., & Moss, S.C. (1996) Mental health problems related to ageing in people with learning disability. In R. Jacoby (Ed.) *A clinical reader in old age psychiatry* . Oxford: Oxford University Press.

3   Patel, P., Goldberg, D.P., & Moss, S.C. (1993) Psychiatric morbidity in older people with moderate and severe learning disability (mental retardation). Part II: The prevalence study. *British Journal of Psychiatry*, 163, 481-491.

4   Moss, S., Prosser H., & Goldberg D. P., (1996) Validity of the schizophrenia diagnosis of the psychiatric assessment schedule for adults with developmental disability (PAS-ADD). *British Journal of Psychiatry*, 168, 359-367.

5   Patel, P., et al (1993) op cit.

6   Moss, S., Goldberg, D., Patel, P. & Wilkin, D. (1993) Physical morbidity in older people with moderate, severe and profound mental handicap, and its relation to psychiatric morbidity. *Social Psychiatry and Psychiatric Epidemiology*, 28, 32-39.

7   Bouras, N., Murray, B, Joyce, T, Kon, Y., & Holt, G. (1995) *Mental Health in Learning Disabilities: A training pack for staff working with people who have a dual diagnosis of mental health needs and learning disabilities*. Brighton: Pavilion.

Further Reading

Bouras, N. (1994) *Mental health in mental retardation*. Cambridge: University Press.

Holland, A., & Moss, S.C. (1996) Mental health problems related to ageing in people with learning disability. In R. Jacoby (Ed.) *A clinical reader in old age psychiatry*. Oxford: University Press.

MENTAL HEALTH SERVICES, RACE AND CULTURE

PRINCIPLES OF SERVICE DELIVERY

Providing mental health services, including the various forms of psychotherapy, to people of racial and ethnic minorities should be based on fairness and on racial and cultural sensitivity. People with similar problems and levels of distress should get the same help in terms of quality, cost, expertise and above all, accessibility and acceptability. The disproportionate numbers of African-Caribbeans in psychiatric hospitals and wards highlight the differences in the way people from different cultures are perceived and treated. Providing culturally sensitive services implies a capacity on the part of purchasers and providers to make appropriate adjustments in service delivery, on the grounds that to ignore factors such as language, different attitudes to gender, racism, social conditions and religious practice would lead to a service that was not adequately meeting the needs of many people.

POSSIBLE UNFAIRNESS AND LACK OF SENSITIVITY

It is the intention of the Department of Health, as expressed in *The Health of the Nation Key Area Handbook in Relation to Mental Illness*[1], that services should be fair to members of different races, and sensitive to cultural practices and values. Policy guidance[2] recommend that purchasers should consider the relevance of services for black and ethnic minority groups when developing contracts. Yet many black people believe the services are actively unfair[3]. The Mental Illness Specific Grant could be used more extensively to develop ethnically sensitive services.

Sources of disquiet lie in a number of places, not least in the views of black professionals working in the field[4]. The following have been identified as causes for concern:

- Firstly, the disproportionate numbers of African-Caribbeans in psychiatric wards, particularly the higher

rates for compulsory detention under *The Mental Health Act, 1983*, for people of African-Caribbean origin[5,6], and also for some people of Asian origins[7]. (On the other hand, earlier studies had not found higher rates of compulsory admissions for patients from Asian "communities").

- Secondly, there have been reports of more compulsory admissions of black patients under the "forensic" sections of *The Mental Health Act, 1983*, and more transfers of patients to secure wards for reasons unconnected with violence[8].

- Thirdly, one study found that people from the Caribbean living in stable families were more likely than whites in similar situations to be admitted to hospital by the police, rather than through GPs[9]. The situation has not been helped by the lack of ethnic monitoring of services[10].

On the whole, lower rates have been found for the admission of people of Asian origins to psychiatric hospitals[11], and lower rates of mental and emotional illness and disorder in the Asian population generally[12], but these findings are not necessarily reassuring. The explanation may be that there are actually lower levels of mental and emotional disorder in the Asian community. But, it is equally possible that the real levels are higher than those recorded and are not adequately recognised and treated. For example, black service users are less likely to be offered psychological therapies or to have access to appropriate preventative services which are culturally acceptable to them. Some evidence also shows that the first contact which people with mental health problems from the Asian community have with services is often the crisis point - leading to compulsory admission.

Black and minority groups believe there is mis-diagnosis, under-diagnosis and over-diagnosis of mental disorder in their communities by psychiatrists. Higher rates for a first diagnosis of schizophrenia have been found among people of

African-Caribbean origins, and many people suspect that such findings are due to psychiatrists' misunderstanding of religious beliefs, or to their failing to appreciate the reasonableness of black people feeling some degree of suspicion towards the white community. Littlewood and Lipsedge[13] expressed the same anxieties. However, Harrison et al.[14] went to considerable lengths to exclude diagnoses made mainly on the grounds of religious belief and "paranoia." The reason for the high levels found in this study has not, so far, been satisfactorily explained. However, racial discrimination, rejection and abuse could well be possible stress factors. Professionals working in this field should always be aware of the possibility that black clients may have had such experiences, and that they have contributed towards their mental health problems. Avoiding the discussion of these issues, because of guilt or fear of hostility, is not a satisfactory solution.

ASPECTS OF ASSESSMENT

A basic requirement for an appropriate mental health service for members of ethnic minorities is that the assessment of needs, both psychiatric and social, be accurate; since a considerable part of intervention and treatment follow from that. A good deal of transcultural psychiatry has been concerned with these issues. Studies have pointed out the dangers of cross-cultural mis-diagnosis, and their consequences in relation to the control and disposal of patients[15, 16]. Their warnings have had some impact. Mental health professionals should neither fail to find mental health problems where they exist, nor "find" them where they do not, for example, by "discovering" psychosis in individuals who may be very distressed, but who, because they hold very different views of the world, become incorrectly labelled as "psychotic" or "schizophrenic". In any case, some psychiatrists and anthropologists would be very suspicious of the World Health Organisation's position[17] that the major categories of Western psychiatry can be applied to people from other cultures, and would prefer to talk about "idioms of distress", which may vary from culture to culture[18].

This debate may be resolved by distinguishing symptoms which are clearly organic and neurological in origin from those that seem heavily influenced by culture, even though they may be expressed largely in physical ways[19]. A rough spectrum could be devised, with at one end, the epileptic-like disorders and the dementias, whose symptoms seem universal, and at the other, anorexia nervosa, bulimia, and "school refusal," which seem to be culture specific. The schizophrenias would be closer to the organic end of the spectrum, although the content of delusions and hallucinations would, of course, be influenced by the client's view of the world, and this, in turn, would be heavily influenced by culture.

In the process of assessment, good communication across any language barrier, and a proper appreciation of social and cultural factors, are necessary for good practice. Even in an interview, the nurse, social worker or doctor must not assume that the conventions about eye contact, proximity and turn taking that apply in his or her own culture apply in another. In addition, good translators, and more importantly, interpreters, who are familiar with the conventions of mental health interviewing, are essential when someone is not fluent in English. Relying on members of the person's family to translate should be avoided since family difficulties may be part of the problem. Obviously, members of the family might well alter the meaning of questions and answers to avoid upsetting their relative - or to save their own embarrassment.

Although the language difficulties of recent Asian immigrants may be easily recognised, it is sometimes assumed that English is the first language of all African-Caribbeans. This is not always the case. For new Caribbean immigrants the first language may be patois. It would not be usual either for Africans to have English as their native tongue.

Culture influences how people experience and express, distress. In some Asian cultures, distress is often expressed physically (somatically) - as we all do to some extent. Voodoo may be part of the belief systems of some racial and ethnic minorities, and clients may be in great distress because they feel they are the victims of hostile magical practices. In some cases, joint assessments with members of a client's ethnic community may help to discover whether particular beliefs or behaviours are part of the person's culture[20].

Activity

- Find out from your local census what proportion of people from different ethnic groups there are in your area.
- Do you think the services in your area adequately address the needs of the ethnic groups represented?

BRITISH BORN CITIZENS AND RECENT IMMIGRANTS

Historically, the relationships between black and white people have been influenced by slavery and colonialism, and this continues to influence the perceptions of many white people even today, so that even when black and Asian people have been born in the UK, they may still be regarded by some people with suspicion or lack of respect.

Although it is assumed that most members of ethnic minorities are not themselves immigrants, in certain communities the rate of immigration is still fairly high. For example, one study found that among a sample of service users from the Pakistani community in a northern town, that more than half of them, and two thirds of the women had entered the UK as adults[21]. Recent immigrants may experience stress not felt by others. For example they may have experienced culture shock by moving not only into a Western culture, but from a peasant to a post-industrial society within a matter of 24 hours[22]. The women in Asian families may be socially isolated, especially if they have entered the UK through arranged marriages, and they have little or no English. For recent immigrants, people who are close to them emotionally may live thousands of miles away, and there may be the stress of separation, nostalgia, abnormal grief when relatives die, and a lack of close confiding relationships[23]. For recent immigrants who are refugees and asylum seekers, there may well be post-traumatic stress disorder as a result of persecution and, increasingly, anxiety due to fear of possible repatriation - a fear which may have intensified due to proposed changes in the immigration laws. As with all ethnic groups, older people may experience additional problems, for example, social isolation may increase due to both general physical problems such as deafness and problems with mobility, and with the experiences of loss and bereavement.

DEALING WITH PEOPLE AS INDIVIDUALS AND AVOIDING STEREOTYPES

Appreciation of the person's culture as a part of understanding his or her situation and predicament is just as important in intervention as in assessment. The client is less likely to engage in treatment where there is a lack of trust. Differences in culture and religion may also create barriers, particularly if the client fears that the worker shows a lack of appreciation and respect for cherished beliefs and values.

Working with any family requires an ability to appreciate the values of that family. Culture affects how behaviour is judged, and may prescribe the status and roles given to family members. Unfortunately, cultural values are often so deeply held that they are hardly discussed. The inexperienced worker may fail to recognise that, for example, to an orthodox Jewish parent, an adolescent child's smoking on the Sabbath may appear almost unforgivable or that in traditional Chinese culture the needs of older people take precedence over the needs of the young[24].

Many members of ethnic minorities may feel that their faith and their own traditional healers have very important parts to play in their recovery of health and well-being, and adopt a twin track approach of consulting their own hakims, priests or rabbis as well as using western medicines. Building up relationships with local community leaders is likely to be an essential part of the job. In addition, traditional Indian remedies may be used as well as western pharmaceuticals, and mental health practitioners need some knowledge of these medicines and their possible side-effects[25].

Most white members of society believe that the mental health services provided try, on the whole, to take into account the values, beliefs and life styles of "British" culture. Services that do not attempt to do this will be regarded as unacceptable. The same should apply to racial and cultural minorities. Appointing ethnic minority professionals would help to increase trust and improve the quality of the service enormously, but, for the foreseeable future, mental health services for people from ethnic minorities will have to be provided largely by the white community. A continuing sensitivity to issues of race and culture is therefore essential to the provision of a quality service. The needs of people with mental health problems from black and ethnic minority groups are often met in a way that is more acceptable to them by services provided by smaller voluntary organisations. These need to be supported and given assistance to develop by statutory services.

Service Example

The "African-Caribbean Mental Health Project" is a Manchester based organisation, which receives funding from a number of sources including the local health authority and social services, the Mental Illness Specific Grant, the Consortium on Volunteering and the King's Fund. The main aims of the project are to:

- *Encourage the relevant and social welfare agencies in the statutory and voluntary sector to become more sensitive, accessible and appropriate to the needs and experiences of the African-Caribbean community in Central Manchester by stimulating debate and discussion and providing information and education.*

- *Facilitate discussion and exploration of mental health issues within the African-Caribbean community*

- *Establish a machinery for dialogue between the community and service providers to enable greater involvement in service planning and delivery.*

- *Provide a direct service which is culturally sensitive and responsive to the needs of individual people in mental distress, their families and carers in both primary and secondary settings.*

- *Promote and support the establishment of self-help and advocacy within the African-Caribbean community aimed at supporting people in maintaining control of their lives and empowering them to discover and follow courses of appropriate action.*

- *To monitor and evaluate its aims and objectives and the work it undertakes to meet them. To ensure that the core purpose remains central to the ACMHP's services and to review its aims accordingly[26].*

• •

DILEMMA

Imran (aged 40) came to the UK in his 20s from Pakistan. He developed schizophrenia in his late 20s but his symptoms have responded well to medication and he no longer needs hospital admissions. Imran lives with his uncle, aunt and their children. The household is rather overcrowded and Imran has shown interest in attending a new day centre in the town.

Day care is arranged for 3 days a week. After two weeks, Imran stops going to the centre, but says the children get him down at home.

You are a worker in the day centre. What issues might you consider?

- There may be a number of reasons why Imran no longer goes to the day care facility. Many service users try a service, but choose to "drop out". Clearly Imran is free to do so.

- Imran may become easily tired on his medication and may not have the energy to take part in activities in the centre.

- Imran may feel reluctant to enter a social group if he doesn't know anyone.

- Is the service sensitive and appropriate to users of Imran's cultural background? Are there any staff or other service users of his nationality/culture? Is the food acceptable?

- Could Imran come with a friend or supporter of his own choice?

- Imran should be supported in saying what he would like/what he dislikes.

What other issues might you consider?

• •

References

1 Department of Health, (1993) *Health of the Nation: Key Area Handbook - Mental Illness.* London: HMSO.

2 Department of Health/SSI (1993) *Caring for People: Mental Illness Specific Grants - monitoring of proposals for use 1992/3.* London: Social Services Inspectorate.

3 Wilson, M. (1993) *Mental Health and Britain's Black Communities.* London: King's Fund.

4 Fernando, S. (ed) (1995) *Mental Health in a Multi-ethnic Society.* London: Routledge.

5 McGovern, D., and Cope, R. (1987) First psychiatric admission rates of first and second generation Afro-Caribbeans. *Social Psychiatry*, 22, 139-149.

6 Barnes, M., Bowl, R. and Fisher, M. (1990) *Sectioned: Social Services and the 1983 Mental Health Act.* London: Routledge.

7 Thomas, C., Stone, K., Osborne, M., Thomas, P. and Fisher M. (1993) Psychiatric morbidity and compulsory admission among UK-born Europeans, Afro-Caribbeans and Asians in Central Manchester. *British Journal of Psychiatry*, 164, 474-480.

8 Cope, R. (1989) The Compulsory Detention of Afro-Caribbeans under the Mental Health Act. *New Community.* 15, (3), 343-356.

9 Ineichen, B., Harrison, G. and Morgan, H.G. (1984) Psychiatric hospital admissions in Bristol. 1. Geographical and Ethnic Factors. *British Journal of Psychiatry.* 145, 600-611.

10 Mental Health Act Commission (1993) *Third Biennial Report, 1987-1989.* London: HMSO.

11 Thomas, C. et al, (1993) op cit.

12 Cochrane, R. and Stopes-Roe, M. (1981) Psychological and social adjustment of Asian immigrants to Britain: a community survey. *Social Psychology*, 12, 195-207.

13 Littlewood, R., and Lipsedge, R. (1982) *Aliens and Alienists.* Harmondsworth: Penguin.

14 Harrison, G., Owens, D. and Holton, A. (1988) A prospective study of severe mental disorder in Afro-Caribbean patients. *Psychological Medicine,* 18, 643-657.

15 Littlewood and Lipsedge (1982) op cit.

16 Rack, P. (1982) *Race, Culture and Mental Disorder.* London: Tavistock.

17 Sartorius, N., Jablensky, A. and Kirten, G. (1986) Early manifestations and first contact incidence of schizophrenia in different cultures. *Psychological Medicine*, 16, 909-928.

18 Kleinman, A., (1987) Anthropology and psychiatry - the role of culture in cross cultural research and illness. *British Journal of Psychiatry.* 151, 447-454

19 Leff, J. (1990) The new "Cross-Cultural Psychiatry" - a case of the baby and the bath water. *British Journal of Psychiatry*, 156, 305-307.

20 Littlewood and Lipsedge (1982) op cit.

21 Hatfield, B., Mohammed, H., Rahim, Z., and Tanweer, H. (1996) Mental Health and the Asian Communities: a local survey. *British Journal of Social Work*, 26, 315-336.

22 Rack, P. (1982) op cit.

23 Hatfield, B. (1996) et al, op cit.

24 Lau, A. (1984) Transcultural Issues in Family Therapy. *Journal of Family Therapy.* 6. 92-112.

25 Rack, P. (1982) op cit.

26 *African-Caribbean Mental Health Project 1995.* Information Sheet

Further Reading

Fernando S. (ed.) (1995) *Mental Health in a Multi-ethnic Society*. London: Routledge.

Rack, P (1982) *Race, Culture and Mental Disorder*. London: Tavistock.

Littlewood R., and Lipsedge R, (1982) *Aliens and Alienists*. Harmondsworth: Penguin

Bandana A. (1990) *Black Perspectives in Social Work*. Birmingham: Ventura Press.

Norman A. (1985) *Triple Jeopardy - Growing Old in a Second Homeland*. London: Centre for Policy on Aging.

Beliappa J. (1991) *Illness or Distress - Alternative Model in Mental Health*. London: Confederation of Indian Organisations.

Webb-Johnson A. (1991) *A Cry for Change - an Asian Perspective in Developing Mental Health Services*. London: Confederation of Indian Organisations.

Good Practices in Mental Health (1995) *Not Just Black and White - An information Pack about Mental Health Services for People from Black Communities*. London: Good Practices in Mental Health.

Department of Health. (1994) *Different Cultures, Different Needs - Video Production*. London: NHS Executive.

• •

This module - "Special Client Groups" - is one of 7 modules in "Learning Materials on Mental Health - an Introduction". The other modules include:

Module 1 - "Recognition of Mental Health Problems"
Module 2 - "Intervention and management"
Module 3 - "Legislation and Guidance"
Module 5 - "Special Issues"
Module 6 - "Users, Carers and Children of Parents with Mental Health Problems"
Module 7 - "Sample Training Exercises"

A sister set of materials is also available for professionals involved in assessing risk - " Learning Materials on Mental Health Risk Assessment"

module

5

SPECIAL
ISSUES

• •

AIMS & OBJECTIVES

After you have worked through this module you should be
better able to:

- Discuss the impact which recent government
  initiatives have had on homeless people with
  mental health problems.

- Identify strategies for managing risk of violence.

- Discuss the impact of substance misuse on people
  with mental health problems.

- Describe key issues involved in assessing and
  managing risk of suicide.

HOMELESS AND MENTALLY ILL PEOPLE

"Individuals have a right to be treated with equal dignity & respect." (Patients Charter Dec. 1991/95)

INCIDENCE OF HOMELESSNESS

Homeless people are often stigmatized by the image of a shambling middle-aged man with a carrier bag in one hand and a bottle in the other! So they are rarely seen as "worthy of respect." Yet the truth is that they come from many different backgrounds and are homeless for many different reasons.

There has been a significant rise in homelessness since 1980. "The numbers doubled between 1980 and 1990, and are still rising."[1]

The visible tip of homelessness represents only a fraction of the picture. The heterogeneous nature, and often high mobility, of homeless people has hampered research into the problem, making it difficult to determine its full significance.

There are many "hidden homeless", sleeping on friends' floors, in squats, or in isolated rural areas.

The old stereotypical picture is belied by recent studies which all show that age and gender vary considerably across different settings. The most notable increase has been in the number of young people who are homeless. "Male hostel residents in Britain are predominantly under 45 years of age, and their mean age has fallen."[2]

Studies have also shown that up to half of mentally disordered remand prisoners have unmet housing needs[3]. Housing difficulties faced by people with mental health problems who have been released from prison include:

- "policies or prejudice from housing providers about criminal records;

- specific conditions/restrictions imposed on discharge (for example, Home Office);

- many seem to have difficulties engaging with services and as a result services may withdraw their help;

- frequent problems of alcohol or drug misuse;

- some individuals with chaotic or rebellious lifestyles may be written off as "uncooperative" and "difficult to manage" by untrained housing mangers;

- specific offences (sexual, violent, arson) are excluded from many forms of housing provision;

- the shortage of high support bedspaces;

- 'nimby-ism' (not in my back yard-ism) and public pressure."[4]

Surveys in recent years have shown that homelessness amongst black and ethnic minority groups was and still is a problem in London, with as many as 43% of people interviewed being from African, African-Caribbean or Asian ethnic groups. These figures are not thought to be representative of areas outside London.[5]

Little direct access provision is culturally sensitive to the particular needs of ethnic minority groups, and often presents an alien and unwelcoming prospect.

Activity

How might you find out how many homeless people there are in your area?

THE IMPACT OF GOVERNMENT POLICIES

Homeless people are entitled to the same health services as the rest of the population, but, for a variety of reasons, they sometimes have difficulty accessing them. Government initiatives have attempted to overcome these difficulties, and funding has been allocated to a number of health authorities specifically to support the provision of services for homeless people.

Other government policies such as the "Rough Sleepers Initiative" and the "Homeless Mentally Ill Initiative" in London, have helped to reduce the numbers sleeping rough in the capital. The Government's aim is to ensure that there is no need for anyone to sleep rough. However concerns still exist among those working with homeless people, "the legislation mentioned in the Queen's speech at the opening of Parliament in 1995 suggests that the Housing Bill currently going through Parliament will, almost certainly, exacerbate the situation."[6]

The Mental Illness Specific Grant could be used in part for social services to develop services for homeless people with mental health problems, for example, having workers to liaise between social services and homeless person's units. There has been wide national variation in the use of the Mental Illness Specific Grant for this purpose.

Under Part III of *The Housing Act, 1985*, local authorities have a legal duty to provide permanent accommodation for those people considered "vulnerable". This category includes, amongst others, people experiencing mental illness.

The new Housing Bill proposes to:

- Remove the automatic rights of homeless people to permanent accommodation.

- Limit the right to temporary accommodation for the "unintentionally homeless" to two years.

- Introduce one year probationary tenancies for new council tenants, allowing badly behaved tenants to be evicted from their homes more easily.[7]

Groups working with homeless people have voiced strong concerns about the possible effects of the bill on vulnerable groups.

PATHWAYS TO HOMELESSNESS

It may be argued that unemployment and stringent housing policies are responsible for the rise of homelessness. The most frequently quoted route into homelessness is, however, through relationship breakdown.[8]

Activity

Consider what effect redundancy and the attendant financial pressures may have on family life and on a person's mental health.

CASE STUDY: Robert

Robert is 43 years old. He had a secure job in the ship-building industry, was married with two children, a mortgage, and a comfortable life-style. With the decline of the ship-building industry, he was made redundant and, despite strenuous efforts, was unable to find other employment.

Robert became depressed and frustrated, unable to cope with his loss of status both in the family and in the wider society. He fell behind with the mortgage repayments and the home was repossessed. Bored, angry and depressed, Robert began to drink heavily. Eventually his wife left him, taking the children with her.

Robert moved into a bed-sit and continued to drink ever more heavily. He was unable to keep up his rent payments and drifted into a transient life-style, often sleeping rough. Ashamed to let them know how he had deteriorated, he lost touch with his family and his old friends.

Now, his only close contact is with other street drinkers. He considers trying to "go dry", but his low self-esteem leads to a fear of failure. He no longer has the confidence to make new friends, find other accommodation or build a new life.

Within the spectrum of mental disorder, incidence of drug and/or alcohol abuse is significantly high, and cases like Robert's are commonplace.

"It is estimated that alcohol misuse in homeless people is three to five times higher than that of the general population"[9] and that drug misuse is becoming more frequent amongst younger hostel users..."[10]

Activity

What difficulties might this create for those providing services for homeless people?

"Alcohol or drugs may help to alleviate depression and boredom. They also help to overcome insomnia in large, noisy hostels, providing a short-term solution to problems."[11]

The breakdown in family relationships also has an adverse effect on young people. Conflict and hostility within a marriage may lead to a young person feeling unable to cope, and running away. This is often true where step-parents are involved.

"Thousands of young, vulnerable people are now homeless. More than 40% of these become homeless after leaving local authority care. Up to 40% of young women who become homeless do so as a result of sexual abuse..."[12]

A large proportion of young, homeless men have also experienced sexual or physical abuse, but are reluctant to disclose the facts. These young people may have no real concept of home or of how to form close, lasting relationships.

HOMELESSNESS AND MENTAL HEALTH PROBLEMS

In view of the emotional trauma experienced by many homeless people it is not surprising that "recent studies suggest that as many as 50% of homeless people suffer some form of mental disorder."[13]

"Individuals, at birth, show physical needs, and, also, in very inchoate form, safety needs...they thrive better when the world shows enough regularity and orderliness so that it can be counted upon..."[14]

What safety is there on the streets? What "regularity and orderliness" is there when people are not sure of a bed for the

night, or food during the day; when there are no facilities available to wash ; or to launder clothes; when there is no privacy; when people have to walk the streets all day with nowhere to shelter?

The urgent and immediate need for warmth, shelter and food, make health issues a low priority for many homeless people. Also, they may feel exposed and ridiculed by other patients, or even GP practice staff, if they do manage to keep appointments at a GP's surgery.

People suffering a variety of illnesses; flu, bronchitis, tuberculosis or even sprained or broken limbs, have no option in some cities but to walk the streets, since direct access hostels and many bed-sits close during the daytime. They learn to ignore their ailments until they become serious enough to require hospital admission or, rather than visit GP surgeries, attend Accident and Emergency departments.

CASE STUDY: John

John is a 58 year old man whose leg became severely ulcerated. Travelling around, and sleeping rough, he was not registered with a GP, nor did he know how to gain access to one, since over years of being alone, he had become severely mentally ill and thought-disordered. It was only when he eventually arrived in an area which did provide good resources for homeless people that his condition was noticed and he was taken into hospital. The leg had to be amputated, but he is still homeless, as he failed to co-operate with his care programme.

PROBLEMS IN ACCESSING SERVICES

"Critics claim that thousands of patients are being discharged into the community as hospitals close due to the government health policy, but that they face inadequate help from local councils and social services."[15] This is thought to be the reason for high levels of mental illness amongst homeless people.

Whilst there may be some truth in this, the accusation that people have been "dumped" as a result of the closure of large psychiatric hospitals is inaccurate. The problem is broader and deeper than this. With the decrease in available bed spaces, the criteria for admission have narrowed. People whose mental health problems are not easily diagnosed may

SUICIDAL BEHAVIOUR

INTRODUCTION

The definition of suicidal behaviour, and particularly that which leads to death, is not straightforward. In general, suicidal behaviour is made up of two separate phenomena, but with a marked degree of overlap between them. In one group are those people who intentionally kill themselves **(suicide)**, or harm themselves intending to end their lives, but who unexpectedly survive **(attempted suicide)**. In the other group are those who intentionally harm themselves, but in the reasonably secure belief that death will not result. This kind of behaviour is often referred to as **"parasuicide"**, because it imitates suicidal behaviour. It is also sometimes referred to as **"deliberate self-harm"**.

With either of these groups it is not difficult to assess suicidal intent, but between these two groups are people whose suicidal motivation will be hard to assess. The person may offer mixed, unclear or shifting ideas when asked about intent, so that it becomes difficult for the professional to assess the seriousness of the action or the risk of repetition. Some episodes of parasuicide have unintended fatal outcomes. On the other hand someone who is determined to commit suicide may survive - and try to conceal continued determination by denying current or future intent. You will see, therefore, that it is possible for an unintended victim to become a fatality and for a potential fatality to become a survivor.

DEMOGRAPHIC AND SOCIAL FACTORS

About 5,000 people kill themselves each year in England, Wales and Scotland[1]. In the USA the figure for suicides is about 30,000. The size of the problem is greater than these figures suggest because many suicides are disguised as accidents or are recorded as "undetermined" deaths. It is estimated that there at least eight to ten suicide attempts for every one completed, but, again, these statistics are unreliable because many attempts go unreported or are concealed by potential victims or those close to them. The reduction of suicide is one of the *Health of a Nation* targets.

Gender

Suicides by men outnumber those by women by a ratio of more than 2:1 but women attempt suicide more often. This may be because depression is more common in women - and depression plays a major role in suicidal behaviour. The greater number of suicides among men reflects the fact that men choose more violent and irreversible methods[2].

Age

In almost all cultures, suicide rises with age. In the UK the highest rates are still found amongst the elderly, in particular those aged over 75, although, in recent years, the rate among men under 45 has risen. In the 15-24 age group suicide has become the second leading cause of death (after "accident"). Young men in prison are almost six times more likely to kill themselves, than those of a similar age outside and 2 per cent of all suicides among men in the 15-44 age group occur in prison. Rates for parasuicide are higher in the younger age groups, particular 15-19, and especially among women (about one in 100 annually). Parasuicide among men peaks between 25-29 years when the annual rate is about one in 200. After the age of 50, the parasuicide rates for both men and women falls to about one in 1000.

Marital status

After standardizing for age and sex, suicide rates are highest in the divorced, followed by the widowed and single. The lowest rates are among married couples.

Social class

In general, suicide and parasuicide rates tend to be higher in the lower social classes, but age is also a significant factor in the social class distribution of suicide. Older people in the highest economic groups are at the highest risk of suicide. The opposite is true for the poorest economic groups, where the 25-44 age group are at highest risk. Higher suicide and parasuicide rates are also significantly correlated with high unemployment[3].

Occupation

Some professional or occupational groups carry a higher risk of suicide than others. For example, vets, pharmacists, dentists, medical practitioners and farmers have higher suicide rates than people in other jobs. One can argue that they all have high levels of stress but they also have access to lethal methods of self-harm, such as drugs, chemicals and firearms.

Ethnicity

Differences among ethnic groups in their suicide rates stem from several factors. Firstly, different cultural attitudes to suicide mean that while some societies regard suicide as unacceptable, others are more tolerant.

Secondly, cultural upheaval may lead to increased levels of stress, particularly among younger people. This can be seen, for instance, among people involved in the major political and social upheaval of the former USSR and parts of Eastern Europe. At another level it can be seen in those ethnic minority groups who are trying to manage and reconcile the clash in standards between their own cultural standards and those of their "host" society. This may be a particular conflict for young people who find themselves, quite literally, caught between two different worlds. Suicide is three times higher than average in young Asian women.

Thirdly, the recognition and treatment of depression reduces the suicide rate. In consequence, rates are likely to be higher in those ethnic and cultural groups where depression goes unnoticed and untreated.

Psychiatric disorders

All categories of psychiatric illness increase the risk of suicide. The highest risk (15%) is among the clinically depressed and alcoholics. For people diagnosed as having schizophrenia, the rate is 10%. Many studies have reported that up to 90% of suicide victims were experiencing a psychiatric disorder at the time of their death. Similar findings have been reported for adolescent suicide victims in

the USA. Mood disorders are most commonly associated with suicide in all age groups. Conduct disorder and depression in childhood also are associated with an increased risk of suicide in adult life.

Repetition

Up to 20% of suicidal people who survive an attempt try again within a year. The mortality rate for parasuicide in the year following an attempt is 1%.

Activity

In your area what services are available for:
- people who have attempted suicide?
- the relatives of people who have committed suicide?

ASSESSMENT

In assessing someone following an episode of parasuicide, we are principally concerned with identifying and assessing elements of "risk". In order to stand the best possible chance of making an accurate assessment of whether the person is at continuing risk, a comprehensive and detailed assessment needs to be undertaken. This is not always easy, because the factual presentation (vague, unreliable or misleading information) and the assessment context (often a busy Accident and Emergency department) are not conducive to achieving good results.

If the person does not speak English then the involvement of a skilled interpreter will be needed in order to make an assessment. Likewise if the person has a communication problem this may need to be addressed, for example, by the use of a signer.

The assessment should cover:

- **Circumstances of episode**: methods used and availability, source of drugs (if used), likelihood of discovery, suicidal communications, motives, precipitants, previous parasuicide episodes; current suicidal thoughts or "hopelessness".

- **Problems and coping strategies**: current problems, worries or anxieties. Particular problems, reflecting "loss" or an anniversary of a suicidal event; evidence of substance dependence or frequent misuse of alcohol or drugs; nature and extent of help-seeking behaviour.

- **Employment record and experiences**: school record of achievement, employment since leaving school, level of skills/ability, periods of unemployment.

- **Social life and activities**: social relationships and recreational activities; degrees of loneliness or social isolation, particularly if language, cultural or ethnic issues seem relevant and important.

- **General health**: previous medical history, psychiatric history and any treatment; current health, especially mood, appetite and sleep.

- **Family structure and relationships**: family of origin; current marital status and family composition; rating of marital relationship and parent/child interaction; emotional climate in the home; frequency of any arguments and history of physical or sexual abuse or neglect.

- **Family circumstances**: environmental problems, low income, housing; family pathology, for example, current or previous crime, psychiatric illness, parasuicide, physical illness/disability; contacts with social agencies.

The assessment must produce at least the minimum amount of information needed to provide the basis for recommendations about the client to be made.

Clearly, the assessor needs good interviewing skills in order to complete a rigourous interview schedule, yet maintain a sensitive pace with a distressed and probably defensive person. With experience, these skills can develop quite quickly but need to be underpinned by the availability of a qualified supervisor.

The risk of someone repeating a suicide attempt, and the possibility of this being fatal, is a continuing concern for professionals in health and social services. Predicting suicide or attempted suicide is difficult, because there are no reliable, discrete predictors. One of the best predictors of completed suicide is a previous attempt, and yet only 1% of people will go on to kill themselves in the following year. The lists of predictors are cumulative, in that the higher the individual score of items, the greater the risk of repetition. This following list is adapted from Kreitman and Foster[4]:

- **previous parasuicide,**

- **diagnosis of personality disorder,**

- **above the recommended maximum levels of alcohol consumption,**

- **previous psychiatric treatment,**

- **unemployment,**

- **Social Class V (the lowest social class)**

- **drug abuse,**

- **criminal convictions,**

- **violence in past five years (perpetrator or victim),**

- **aged 25-54 years,**

- **single, widowed or divorced.**

Kreitman and Foster found that patients scoring positively on three or fewer of the above listed items had a repetition rate of 4.9%. For those scoring between four and seven items, the rate was 20.5%. For those scoring eight or more, the repetition rate went up to 41.5%. In all but the lowest scoring group, men had increasingly higher repetition rates than women. There is a real problem of "specificity" in studies of this kind, because not only do they identify successfully those repeaters who have "high" risk scores, but they identify a great many "false positives" - non-repeaters with high scores. Nearly 60% in Kreitman and Foster's study scored eight or more items, but did not repeat parasuicide. Predictive scales are, therefore, of more value when used with large groups, but continuing research will help to refine their sensitivity. It is arguably of more value to a person, if risk factors raise the level of concern, which then influence the formulation of management plans, rather than diverting professionals into making predictions. All suicidal behaviour is cause for concern, but where demand greatly exceeds the availability of therapeutic resources, a system of matching interventions to "high", "medium" or "low" levels of risk may help to reduce pressure on resources to more manageable levels.

MANAGEMENT

The management of suicidal people is clearly related to the degree of risk and a comprehensive assessment provides valuable information. Using a risk list, it is possible to suggest actions or activities to help the person to "recover" from the episode, achieve a reasonable level of satisfaction with their family and friends, and provide safeguards against further suicidal behaviour.

- **"Mild" Risk** - At the "mild" end of the spectrum, counselling to help them to express their feelings of despair and hopelessness, and suicidal thoughts, will also help to clarify any problems responsible for those feelings. Linking the person with sources of help and advice, and helping them to develop or improve problem-solving skills, is likely to be beneficial.

- **"Moderate" Risk** - People assessed as being at "moderate" risk may need similar help to those at the "low" level , but will also need closer monitoring and supervision, together with psychiatric assessment and possibly treatment. Given adequate resources, people at "moderate" risk can be maintained very effectively in the community, but they may need to be admitted to hospital if there is a significant increase in risk.

- **"High" Risk** - The "high" risk person must go into hospital either on a voluntary or compulsory basis. Even in hospital, the "high" risk patient needs regular, possibly constant, surveillance, until there is sustained improvement in their mental state.

Whatever the level of assessed risk, it is the capacity of the worker to spend time with the person, providing the individual with opportunities and encouragement to talk about his or her distress and despair, that leads to recovery. Careful and skilful interviewing usually uncovers any residual suicidal risk, even though, for example, the person may be making a good recovery from depression. Individual and family methods of treatment have been used very effectively with suicidal people. Developing skills in problem-solving, stress management, and communication are usually prominent features of these forms of treatment. Accessing and mobilising family and community supports are important.

● ●

DILEMMA

Janet is 48 years old and lives alone. Her husband left her 20 years ago after the birth of their daughter Clara. Clara now lives locally and holds a spare key to Janet's home.

Janet suffers from epilepsy and has experienced depression for the past two years . During this period she has expressed clear suicidal thoughts and has been admitted to hospital on two separate occasions. She was discharged from hospital last month and has been receiving regular visits from support staff since. Recently Janet appears to be feeling increasingly negative.

You (a support worker) visit one morning at an arranged time and find that you can't get an answer when you ring the doorbell. This is unusual for Janet, although it has happened on a previous occasion when she had "popped out" to see her neighbour. You 'phone her daughter, but there is no reply. You are unhappy with the situation and do not feel that it would not be appropriate to leave and return again later.

What might you do?

- Check with the neighbours to find out when she was last seen (ensuring that you maintain Janet's confidentiality).

- Try 'phoning; she may not answer the door, but she might answer the 'phone, particularly if you let it ring persistently.

- Find out from the last support worker who visited whether Janet had indicated any reason why she couldn't make the arranged time.

- Ask this support worker what Janet's mental state was like on the last visit.

MODULE 5

- Report to the care manager the problems you are having in gaining access to the house. Pass on any relevant details you have discovered from other support staff regarding Janet's mental state.

- The care manager should then try to gain access once again.

- If this is not possible the care manager may decide to contact the police with a view to forcing entry. If the situation is considered a mental health emergency, a warrant will be required to gain entry to the property - it is the responsibility of the ASW to arrange this.

Clearly the action taken by the support worker will depend on how serious he/she believes the situation is. It is important that decisions are taken quickly. For example, in a situation of overdose, intervention is essential within a short period of time.

Can you think of any alternative courses of action you might have taken?

How might the situation have been prevented in the first place?

● ●

References

1   Charlton, J., Kelly, S., Dunnell, K., Evans, B., and Jenkins, R., (1993) Suicide deaths in England and Wales: trends in factors associated with suicide deaths. *Population Trends.* 71. 34-42.

2   Charlton, J., Kelly, S., Dunnell, K., Evans, B., Jenkins, R., and Wallis, R., (1992) Trends in suicide deaths in England and Wales. *Population Trends.* 69. 10-16.

3   Platt, S and Kreitman, N. (1984) Trends in parasuicide and unemployment among men in Edinburgh 1968-82. *British Medical Journal.* 289. 1029-1032.

4   Kreitman, N and Foster, J., (1991) The construction and selection of predictive scales with particular reference to parasuicide. *British Journal of Psychiatry.* 159. 185 - 192.

Further Reading

Jenkins, R., Griffiths, S., Wylie, I., Hawton, K., Morgan, G., and Tylee, A (Eds) (1994) *The Prevention of Suicide.* London: HMSO.

Health Advisory Service (1994) *Suicide Prevention: The Challenge Confronted.* London: HMSO.

Department of Health. (1994) *Health of the Nation: Key Area Handbook - Mental Illness.* Second edition. London: HMSO.

● ●

This module - "Special Issues" - is one of 7 modules in "Learning Materials on Mental Health - An Introduction". The other modules include:

Module 1 - "Recognition of Mental Health Problems"
Module 2 - "Intervention and Management"
Module 3 - "Legislation and Guidance"
Module 4 - "Special Groups"
Module 6 - "Users, Carers and Children of Parents with Mental Health Problems"
Module 7 - "Sample Training Exercises"

A sister set of materials is also available for professionals involved in assessing risk - "Learning Materials on Mental Health Risk Assessment"

module 6

SERVICE USERS, CARERS, AND CHILDREN OF PARENTS WITH MENTAL HEALTH PROBLEMS

AIMS & OBJECTIVES

After you have worked through this module you should be better able to:

- Discuss the importance of users' views in the development of mental health services.
- Identify the methods by which users can be encouraged to participate
- Describe the consequences which caring for a person with a mental illness may have on the carer's life.
- Identify factors which may alleviate stress for carers.
- Discuss the impact which a parent's mental illness may have on a child.
- Identify the services needed for the children of mentally ill parents

USERS

USER OR CONSUMER?

Many different terms are used to describe people who receive help from mental health professionals. We have to be careful to be precise about our terminology so that we can be confident that we are talking about the same thing. The term "service user" is often employed. In this sense a "user" can mean anyone who has contact with psychiatric services, or anyone who has seen a psychiatrist. The Care Programme Approach requires users to be involved in the planning of their own care (see Modules 2 and 3). In the CPA, a user is someone who has contact with psychiatric services. Some health service providers choose to interpret "psychiatric services" narrowly, to mean only those people who are in contact with statutory services (usually with a psychiatrist) and some interpret it more widely to include all mental health service agencies, professionals and voluntary groups.

The term "survivor" is not without difficulty. It implies that people have survived psychiatric treatment, and while some ex-patients do talk about their care in this way, most do not. A more positive interpretation of the term "survivor" is that it means surviving a mental health system which eroded confidence and dignity, and surviving the difficult life experiences which led to the need for mental health care.

Users of psychiatric services are often referred to as "consumers". The appropriateness of this term depends on the extent to which mental health services have the five essential features of consumerism:

- **Access** - what services are offered to whom; how easy they are to use: where they are ; when they are available.

- **Choice** - consumers influence services; users' interests are considered; their views are part of monitoring the services.

- **Information** - consumers are fully informed about services; providers seek out and react to information from users.

- **Redress** - clear and efficient complaint procedures exist and are publicised; consumer feedback is used to make changes.

- **Representation** - users' views are sought and made known to help make decisions; voluntary organisations are consulted; there is a system of advocacy[1].

By giving service users more choice and by making mental health services which have the features of consumerism, we do treat them more like consumers. In mental health care it is not always possible to give the consumer choice, and in some circumstances we have to remove their freedom to choose and admit them to hospital against their wishes. Some interpretations of liberty and freedom lead to the rejection of all forms of compulsory treatment. Not all ex-patients would accept this. About two-thirds of ex-patients (asked when they are well) think that the use of pressure and force is justified sometimes. Most ex-patients agree that treatment can be refused, except in a psychiatric emergency. Given the choice (when well) most ex-patients will advise their service providers to use compulsion in an emergency if they become unwell again[2].

This debate raises several points:

1. The user movement contains many disparate and sometimes opposing views.

2. Organisations which claim to speak on behalf of a particular group should be clear that the views they express are widely held.

3. Anyone proposing to represent user views must base his or her case on evidence gained by careful listening to what is actually being said. This applies to all organisations, including the health service.

Representativeness

How representative are "user views"? This question has hampered the development of user involvement. One could say that any user is "representative" of users, but at the same time not all service users are able to, or wish to, represent others' views. It has been said that there are as many views as there are users[3]. In a representative democracy, elected representatives are expected to seek out and reflect the views of their constituents. Speaking directly for oneself is participative, rather than representative, democracy. The legitimacy of the participating user lies in personal experience - and all personal experiences are valid. It may be unrealistic to expect users representatives to report back to the whole of their constituency - all other users of that service. Users who participate as a representative for a long time, are different from people new to user status. Paradoxically, they can become less "representative" by being more accomplished in acting as a user representative. However, it can be argued that they gain in influence as a result of this enhanced status and their participation is more effective.

WHAT DO WE NEED TO PROVIDE TO INVOLVE USERS MORE?

Broadly speaking, we need to provide information and opportunities for participation.

Information

Several channels for feedback from users already exist in the NHS[4]:

- direct personal contact;

- consumer choice;

- making a complaint;

- patient advocates;

- patient representative groups;

- community development projects in health;

- observation by NHS managers;

- local patient sample surveys;

- Community Health Council intervention;

- health board members;

- local and national media reports and campaigns;

- academic research;

- national pressure group activity; and

- general elections(!).

Acivity

Look at the list of NHS "feedback channels" identified above.
- How are they used in relation to people with mental health problems?
- How could feedback be improved?

Participation

One way of improving involvement is to establish a dialogue between the health commissioners (District Health Authority), the personal social services and local people. It is important to explore ways in which consumers can improve and increase their ability to influence the planning and delivery of health care. Of central importance are: the development of two-way communication between consumers and professionals; and giving attention to the way consumers are supported to develop their involvement[5]. The lessons from our experience to date include:

- organisational change in health services is often undertaken with insufficient consideration of the views of users and other interested parties;

- it may be unwise and inappropriate to develop consumer expectations of participation in the absence of adequate support (such as health authority resources and staff time);

- the sort of skills needed for dialogue between the services and the users are: knowledge of the community, listening skills and going at the respondent's pace; these need to be in place at the outset of the planning and development process;

- the process of consultation is time consuming (8-15 hours a week for every location);

- material collected from informal meetings and in an informal way is difficult to collate;

- GPs often think that liaison with local community groups is relatively unimportant;

- GPs are reluctant to get involved in planning with groups containing patients outside their practice;

- people are usually pleased to be asked about health issues; and

- professionals have heavy caseloads which means that they are often unable to give priority to planning new developments and to local group meetings with users.

INFORMATION ABOUT TREATMENT PROGRAMMES

MIND[6] suggests that user information about care and treatment programmes should cover:

- diagnosis;

- services people can expect from an authority;

- alternative treatments;

- expected side-effects;

- how to complain; and

- access to health records.

Consumer satisfaction surveys are a common source of information about the impact of a mental health programme. They are now commonplace in the NHS, as are clinical audits. But these are not often able to answer the question about the user's experience. "Consumer audit" is the term for gathering user's information by focus groups, observation, and home interviews. The content looks at the health service from the users' point of view and assesses its quality. A multi-method approach is preferable and questionnaires alone are likely to miss the complexity and ambivalence of users' relations with mental health services[7].

The development of unique research methods to assess satisfaction in each service makes comparison between services impossible, but this might be offset by the greater detail and understanding which is obtained from specific assessments of satisfaction. It is likely that both systematic and standardised assessments should be combined with more detailed specific enquiries in order to obtain a complete picture.

INFORMATION AT THE PERSONAL LEVEL

It has been suggested that services should deal with their most obvious problems, before setting up user feedback mechanisms[8]. The arguments are:

- obvious problems can be addressed quickly and one does not waste users' time and energy identifying problems which are already known;

- if providers are seen to be doing something positive, then users will take them more seriously and may think involvement is more worthwhile;

- staff need to face the challenge of change before they can make best use of user opinion; and

- suggested improvements coming first from users can make services defensive, and lead to user feedback being marginalised.

PARTICIPATION IN TREATMENT PROGRAMMES

There is a need for a good practice guide to involving consumers in meetings[9]. Many of the users of mental health services are sensitive to the interpersonal or public nature of meetings. Indeed, their problems may even have started there, resulting in, say, withdrawal from social gatherings, and anxiety or even panic in public places. Nevertheless, the following guidance may be useful to those wishing to consider user involvement in aspects of what we provide in the mental health programme, be it a day centre, a drop-in or a clinic.

Important issues are: access, information, communication, power, and group dynamics. New members do not share the interpersonal history of the group they are joining, but eventually they become part of it. Access is an important issue, involving:

- transport and finance problems;
- choice of venue and time;
- expenses;
- fees (which raises earnings/union issues);
- language; and
- the lack of administrative support.

When training or introducing new group members it is important to:

- avoid jargon;
- provide an agenda and minutes in advance;
- recognise that users are also experts in some things, and
- provide background information (professionals often treat new professionals worse than users in this respect).

It has been suggested that information should also be provided about the reasons why people are invited to participate in the meeting[10].

Consider also:

- the length of meetings;
- time for people to study and receive comments on consultation documents;
- the provision of funds for users to buy in the help they need (which has an extra benefit over providing the help in kind - by permitting greater user choice[11]); and
- the provision of help in kind, such as photocopying, meeting rooms, access to training and so on. (One might also add to this list resources for: message-handling, typing, secretarial services and phone calls. Funding for attendance payments, respite care and hotel accommodation would also be helpful).

• •

DILEMMA

A joint care planning team was established in your area. Over the course of the first nine months, "users" were represented by Sarah, who had a history of manic depression. Sarah generally contributed very little to the meetings. When she became ill, Sarah withdrew from the meetings completely. At the following meeting she was replaced by another female service user, Halina. Halina attended two meetings and became quite involved in discussions. After the last meeting, however, Halina telephoned the team coordinator and informed him that she found the meetings extremely stressful and no longer wanted to be involved.

What issues about the arrangement of user representation does this dilemma suggest to you?

- Are the meetings perhaps too "powerful"?
- Is there too much use of jargon?
- There may be an element of "tokenism" - "we've got a user on our sub-committee!"

What other issues might you consider?

What steps might you suggest to deal with these issues?

- The meetings might be less intimidating if there were two service users involved.

- Perhaps the format of the meeting could be changed so that it is less formal.

- It might be useful for one of the professionals involved to attend the users own meeting.

What other steps might you consider?

● ●

PARTICIPATION AT THE INDIVIDUAL LEVEL

At this level the main involvement will be in the individual care plan. The Care Programme Approach (see Modules 2 & 3) should eventually ensure that user and carer involvement in the assessment, care planning and review becomes a reality. This is one area in which the interests of users and carers may differ, since the care plans are for the user, not the carer, and the former may not want the latter to be involved in the process. The assessment of carers' needs has become mandatory from April 1996. Previously the *Disabled Persons Act ,1986,* required carers' views to be taken into account.

Another aspect of involvement at the individual level is in users' self-assessment. This, as opposed to or perhaps in addition to professional assessment, can be expected to be used more. User-ratings of their own quality of life is a central aspect of the *Lancashire Quality of Life Profile*[12] and self-assessment of this sort will be used alongside other forms of quality assurance. Users in some services have been trained to make quality of life assessments. User participation in evaluation can also be expected to develop in the future in a number of ways, for example:

- as subjects;

- as consumers of research findings;

- as facilitators between the community and the evaluation agency;

- in project planning groups;

- and acting as independent evaluators.

Useful addresses

**Nottingham Advocacy Group
and Nottingham Patient's Council Support Group,**
9A Forest Road East,
Nottingham, NG1 4HJ
(0115)-9484111.

Survivors Speak Out
34 Osnaburgh Street,
London NW1 3ND
0171 916 5472/3.

UK Advocacy Network (UKAN)
Suite 417, Premier House,
14 Cross Burgess Street,
Sheffield S1 2HG
(0114) 2753131.

Breakthrough
8 Trevelyan Place,
Crook,
County Durham DL15 9UY

References

1   *Consumer Involvement Project* (CIP) (1994) Wiltshire Health Authority, Devizes, Wiltshire.

2   Luckstead, A. and Coursey, R.D. (1995) Consumer perceptions of pressure and force in psychiatric treatments. *Psychiatric Services* 46(2):146-152.

3   Strong, S. (1995) *Work and Training: Draft literature review.* Prepared for the Sainsbury Centre for Mental Health Work and Training Working Group.

4   Jones, L. Leneman, L. and Maclean, U. (1987) *Consumer Feedback for the NHS: A literature review,* London: King's Fund.

5   Consumer Involvement Project (CIP) (1994) op.cit.

6   MIND (1991) *MIND's Policy on User Involvement.* London: MIND.

MODULE 6

7   Mangen, S. and Griffith J. (1982) Patient satisfaction with
    community psychiatric nursing: a prospective controlled
    study. *J.Adv.Nursing* 7:477-482.

8   Robbins, S. (1993) *Users views - From a provider's
    viewpoint.* In R. Leiper and V.Field (eds) *Counting for
    Something in Mental Health.* Aldershot: Avebury.

9   Consumer Involvement Project (CIP) (1994) op.cit.

10 Lindow, V. and Morris, J. (1995) *Service user
    involvement.* Joseph Rowntree Foundation.

11 Goss, S. and Miller C. (1995) *From Margin to
    Mainstream: Developing user- and carer- centred
    community care.* Joseph Rowntree Foundation and
    Community Care.

12 Oliver, J.P.J., Huxley, P.J., Bridges, K. & Mohamad, H.
    (1996) *Quality of Life and Mental Health Services.*
    London: Routledge.

Further Reading

Barnes, M. Cormie, J. and Crichton, M. (1994) *Seeking
representative views from frail older people.* Scotland: Age
Concern.

Clarke, S. (1994) *Obtaining Consumer Views - Qualitative and
Quantitative Methods.* Consumer Involvement Project (CIP)
(1994) The Health Commission for Wiltshire and Bath,
Devizes, Wiltshire.

Consumer Involvement Project (CIP) Leaflet available from -
Wiltshire Health Authority, Communications Department,
Southgate House, Pans lane, Devizes. SN10 5EQ.

Leiper, R. and Field, V. (eds) (1993) *Counting for Something
in Mental Health.* Aldershot: Avebury.

UKAN (United Kingdom Advocacy Network) (1994) *Advocacy
- A Code of Practice.* NHS Executive Mental Health Task Force
User Group.

CARERS

MODULE 6

"To enable users and carers to exercise genuine choice and participate in the assessment of their care needs and in the making of arrangements for meeting those needs, local authorities should publish readily accessible information about their care services.

Departments should identify what arrangements they intend to make to inform users and carers about services."[1]

INTRODUCTION

In the community, psychiatric patients with long-term problems are often separated from their families and have limited support. However, it is important to remember that when they first become ill, most people with mental health problems are living with their family. Almost two-thirds of people diagnosed with schizophrenia for the first time live with their families. About half of adult mentally ill people live in families with children.

Carers have needs quite distinct from those of users of services. The involvement of carers in mental health services is similar to the need to involve those people using the services. The constraints on them creating their own organisations are similar and both have to deal with the same health and social services bureaucracy. Carers become involved in mental health services in order to improve them for the users as well as for themselves.

We know that carers, especially those coping with relatives with more severe disorders, experience stress, poor health and financial demands[2, 3]. The most vulnerable carers lack material and social resources. They may have unrealistic expectations for the support of their relative. In addition, they are unlikely to gain much pleasure from the tasks of caring and may have limited coping skills compared to less vulnerable carers. Successful work with carers pays attention to their specific needs, and looks at the results of help as well as the processes.

TERMINOLOGY

Early work referred almost exclusively to the burden of mental illness for carers. Later, it was suggested that this was inappropriate and that the more neutral term, the "need for support", should be used instead. Some people suggested that the term "family impact" might be better[4, 5], but this term has given way to the desire to consider a term which reflects the positive aspects of living with a mentally ill relative. Accordingly, the term "family caregiving" is becoming more widely accepted. Referring to the main source of informal support to the patient as the "caregiver" emphasises the positive, desirable aspects of the process rather than the negative ones. The needs of children who care for their mentally ill parents are now gaining attention. They have special needs. The sort of support they need differs from that provided to adult caregivers, whose average age is likely to be about 40 or older. Children who are caregivers may experience developmental problems, which adversely affect their self-image and self esteem[6].

(For further information on Children of Mentally Ill Parents, refer to page 143)

THE EXPERIENCE OF DIFFERENT GROUPS

In the literature on carers, people caring for a mentally ill relative tend to receive less attention than other carers, in spite of the fact that the burden of caring for a mentally ill relative is probably greater. There is insufficient research for us to know the exact pattern of differences in the experience of caring for people with different illnesses, for example, dementia, schizophrenia, depression.

However, research on dementia shows:

- 90% of the carers of people diagnosed as having dementia feel restricted in some way and 40% have minor mental health difficulties[7].

- Lack of carer well-being is particularly associated with incontinence, disturbance at night and the need for constant supervision among people with dementia[8].

- Reported problems and stress in carers are associated with more severe illnesses, whereas passive behavioural problems, such as apathy, are better tolerated by the dementia group[9, 10].

The absence of behavioural problems may be associated with well-being and the success of community care. Among both older and mentally ill people, a key indicator of the need for care is the person's inability to deal with the activities of daily living. This evidence suggests that carers of people with severe mental illness find clients' deficiencies in daily living skills, behavioural problems and need for constant attention the major sources of stress. It is hardly surprising that, in general, about three-quarters of the relatives of people with mental illnesses show symptoms of psychological or physical ill-health[11]. Help in these specific areas, which are worse the more the person experiences the negative symptoms of schizophrenia or depression, is likely to bring relief to the caregiver.

· ·

DILEMMA

Your community mental health team receive a letter from a carer indicating that the carer support group to which she belongs feel that your team do not adequately meet the needs of carers. The writer asks for a meeting to discuss carers needs in general and the needs of the group in particular.

What issues might you expect to arise and how might you handle them?

Issues which might arise

- Lack of information about services/medication, how to deal with symptoms/behaviour and so on.

- Carers often feel that they are not being listened to and they may feel that the team are unaware of the tasks, burden and distress which they face as carers.

- The carers may feel that they are excluded from decisions and that communication between professionals and carers is poor. For example, in relation to the planning of services when a client is discharged from hospital.

- The carers may feel that your team or services are inaccessible for carers.

- The carers may feel they receive conflicting information and that they cannot get to speak with the same person twice.

- The poor physical and mental health of carers

- Carers often have financial difficulties and are socially isolated.

- Ageing carers may be concerned about what will happen to their relative when they can no longer care for them.

- The carers may be dissatisfied with the limited resources available.

What other issues might arise?

How the issues might be handled

- Any means of providing carers with additional information should be explored - for example, the production of an information leaflet on services and benefits.

- A representative from your team could arrange to attend the carers' group meetings.

- To avoid the problem of carers receiving conflicting or inadequate information, the carers need a long term commitment by a professional who they can develop a good working relationship with and who will carry out routine assessments and reviews of their needs as well as the service users'.

- Regular visits by a professional to offer emotional support and discuss problems.

- The carers' needs should be assessed and reviewed on a regular basis.

- Your team could consider appropriate ways of finding out the views of all carers using your services. The results obtained could be used to set standards for the team to work towards in the future.

In what other ways could the issues raised be handled?

● ●

TYPES AND SOURCES OF STRESS FOR CAREGIVERS

The sources of stress for caregivers come from the material and emotional impact of the illness on the household. Some people are more vulnerable to stress when providing care, and caregiving for a mentally ill person may have some particularly stressful features. (Both of these points are dealt with later).

Material problems

One study found that a quarter of a sample of discharged patients had leisure, money, and work problems[12]. In 60% of cases, the carer's social relationships had been adversely affected. However, for some of the carers, personal relationships became more important to them as a result of the illness and they felt that their "values changed for the better". In many cases carers find that they spend more time in their own home and so their own social life becomes seriously restricted and disrupted. Children in families of a mentally ill person tend to participate in fewer out-of-school activities.

If carers continue to work, then their performance at work may suffer. In many cases, the carer has to take time off work or give up work altogether, with serious financial consequences. One estimate suggests that almost 40% of carers have financial problems and 80% feel that their financial situation has been adversely affected[13].

Hardly any studies have been able to demonstrate a real improvement in the material circumstances of carers. This could be because the interventions which were used were not powerful enough to produce a change in the carer's quality of life. A study of Family Support Workers (FSWs) showed that the quality of life of newly referred carers was worse in some respects than the quality of life of carers who had been receiving FSW support[14].

Emotional responses

The most lucid accounts of caregiving and its impact tend to be about the emotional aspects. An "Involvement Evaluation Questionnaire" has been developed to measure these aspects. It is divided into: tension; supervision; worrying; and urging. It also includes a specific distress scale and asks about the care of children. About half of carers can experience constant worry[15]. Other common experiences are:

- being unsure whether to prompt the relative into activity or to allow withdrawal;

- feeling frustrated and baffled;

- being upset about being embarrassed in public;

- often feeling like one is living with a completely different person;

- marital conflict in cases of depression;

- fear of the patient;

- fear for the future;

- anger and resentment;

- resignation.

The most common feeling is of being overloaded. Uncertainty is extremely common. Most mental illnesses are fluctuating conditions and the carers find themselves watching for signs of recurrence. In this respect, mental illness is unlike physical disability which begins in childhood, or progressive disorders. As well as these generally negative emotional experiences, many carers report positive emotions of warmth and love towards their relative.

The adverse impact on physical and mental health tends to be higher in new cases, perhaps because the early experience is more traumatic and involves the loss of stability, and the loss of the known and loved "person". The impact of mental illness seems to differ according to the socio-economic group, gender, race and age of the carer, as well as the level of social support available, but there is less definitive research in these areas.

THE CARING TASK AND VULNERABLE CARERS

It is essential to provide practical help to families with a member who is physically disabled; with a mental illness it tends to be different in that the carer is usually responsible in ways not always so tangible. These might include:

- supervising medication;

- managing problem behaviour;

- overseeing household and personal care.

This is often undertaken for a relative who is reluctant to be helped and reluctant to cooperate.

The negative problems experienced by a mentally ill person - the lack of abilities, the desire to withdraw, the absence of motivation and the neglect of self - are the hardest things for carers to live with. In depressed patients the most difficult

aspects are: threatened or attempted suicide ; withdrawal and no inclination to speak; and hypochondriacal thoughts.

Carers who appear to be the most vulnerable to these stresses are those who have:

- **fewer material and social resources;**

- **unrealistic expectations;**

- **limited or poor coping skills;**

- **fewer rewards from the caring process.**

THE VALUE OF PSYCHOSOCIAL INTERVENTIONS

The influence of early work, which suggested that families caused schizophrenia has rightly disappeared. There is a great deal of research, however, which suggests that relatives' levels of expressed hostility and emotion ("expressed emotion") do affect relapse rates (see Module 1). A lot of work has been done on training programmes, which enable mental health staff to improve the situation in such families.

A number of studies have suggested that psychosocial interventions may be helpful in reducing the adverse aspects of caregiving. Positive changes in carer distress, subjective burden and coping have been found[16]. Prognosis tends to be unfavourable where there are high levels of hostile and critical remarks, referred to as "expressed emotion". This causes relapse in schizophrenia, especially when the person is not protected from the effects by medication and less face-to-face contact.

In treatment studies psychosocial interventions have been shown to have positive effects[17]. One study found that brief counselling helped caregivers only modestly[18], and it was suggested that such help would have greater impact if the worker doing the counselling was the carer's primary worker, while still being a member of the multidisciplinary team working with the client. This is the model of care used by the Making Space family support workers and was felt to be a key variable in a better outcome for carers.

WHAT SORT OF SERVICES CARERS VALUE

There appears to be agreement about how services can meet carers' needs. Greater levels of distress have been found in those receiving no social or medical support[19]. In many instances carers have substantial unsatisfied needs[20]. Most unresolved problems appear to be associated with the emotional aspects of caregiving.

Among the features which make life difficult for carers are:

• frequent staff changes;

• the failure to intervene early in a deteriorating situation; and

• the lack of a positive attitude to the carer's problems.

Carers' needs should be considered from the first contact with the service. This is now being written into the legislation (see *The Care Programme Approach, 1990*; and *The Carers (Recognition and Services) Act, 1995).* This gives carers, who are providing substantial care on a regular basis, the right to request their own assessment at the time of the user's assessment[21].

Carers' problems may be reduced by:

• close cooperation between the carer and professionals;

• information and advice;

• day care;

• flexible packages of care - including agreed participation in the client's Care Programme Approach;

• care for their own needs;

• periods of respite;

• services which support clients at home.

The impact on carers of the type of mental health services provided has been studied. The results have been mixed and have not, to date, shown major improvements in carer well-being[22]. Brief care produced more distress than standard care at two weeks (because of the slowness of recovery of the patient) and at 14 weeks (because of patient dependence). Standard care produced more distress regarding the impact on family employment at two weeks, and at 14 weeks more distress regarding the carer's own leisure activities and social life.

In another comparison of a standard service with a comprehensive community service, the impact on the carer was reduced in both services due to improved client behaviour[23]. Only the comprehensive community service improved the carers' feelings about the clients' social performance. Neither the standard nor the comprehensive services changed the carers' material circumstances. There is clearly a need for more research into successful interventions which help carers. Extending the care programme and care management arrangements to carers might help the carer and the service user.

Activity

Some key issues to resolve - consider how to:

• provide for hidden groups of carers, for example in minority ethnic groups, or children who are carers.

• ensure that different carer groups are adequately represented in consultation sessions, or have people who can speak for them.

• recognise and manage situations in which the interests of the carer and the user are not identical.

• recognise and assimilate the fact that the carer's capacity to care will vary over time, and listen for indications that this is happening.

• involve carers in assessments and in the care planning process.

• monitor the implementation of a joint health and social services strategy for carers.

• use specific allocations of government funding to create services for carers which will meet their needs.

References

1   *Community Care in the next decade and beyond: Policy Guidance.* London: HMSO (1990 (3.18) & (2.25)

2   Kahana, E.Biegel, D.E., and Wykle, M.L. (1994) *Family Caregiving Across the Lifespan*, California: Sage.

3   Schulz, R. and Williamson, G.M. (1993) Psychosocial and behavioural dimensions of physical frailty. *Journal of Gerontology* 43:39-43.

4   Perring, C., Twigg, J. and Atkin, K. (1990) *Families caring for people diagnosed as mentally ill: the literature reexamined.* York: SPRU.

5   Sorenson, T. and Grunnvold, O. (1994) *The Norwegian Family Impact Questionnaire.* University of Oslo, Psychiatric Department, Ulleval Hospital Oslo, Norway.

6   Aldridge, J. and Becker, S. (1993) *Children who care - inside the world of young carers.* Loughborough: Loughborough University.

7   Levin, E., Moriarty, J. and Gorbach, P. (1994) *Better for the Break.* NISW, London: HMSO.

8   Levin, E., Sinclair, I. and Gorbach, P. (1989) *Families, Services and Confusion in Old Age.* Aldershot: Gower.

9   Burns, A., Jacoby, R. and Levy, R. (1990) Psychiatric phenomena in Alzheimer's disease iv: Disorders of behaviour *British Journal of Psychiatry* 157:86-94.

10 O'Connor et al (1990) Problems reported by relatives in a community study of dementia. *British Journal of Psychiatry* 156:835-41.

11 Gibbons, J.S., Horn, S.M., Powell, JM et al (1984) Schizophrenic patients and their families: a survey in a psychiatric service based on a DGH unit *British Journal of Psychiatry* 144:70-77.

12 Stengard, E. and Salokangas R.K.R. (1994) *Living with the mentally ill.* Department of Public Health, University of Tampere, Finland.

13 Gibbons, J.S., et al, op.cit.

14 Making Space (1995) *Making More Space: The Unique and Vital Contribution of the Family Support Worker.* Making Space, Warrington; MHSWRU, Manchester University.

15 Stengard, E. and Salokangas R.K.R. op.cit.

16 Falloon, I. and Pederson, J. (1985) Family management in the prevention of morbidity of schizophrenia: the adjustment of the family unit. *British Journal of Psychiatry.* 147:156-63.

17 Brooker, C. Tarrier, N., Barrowclough, C. et al (1992) Training Community Psychiatric Nurses for psychosocial interventions: Report of a pilot study. *British Journal of Psychiatry* 160:836-844.

18 Szmukler, G.I., Herrman, H., Colusa, S. et al (in press) A controlled trial of a counselling intervention for caregivers of relatives with schizophrenia. *Social Psychiatry and Psychiatric Epidemiology.*

19 Johnstone, E.C, Owens, D.G.C, Gold, A. et al (1984) Schizophrenic patients discharged from hospital - a follow-up study. *British Journal of Psychiatry* 145:586-590.

20 Creer, C. and Wing, J.K. (1974) *Schizophrenia at home.* Surbiton: National Schizophrenia Fellowship.

21 Carer's (Recognition and Services) Act 1995. *Policy Guidance and Practice Guide.* London: HMSO.

22 Platt, S. and Hirsch, S. (1981) The effects of brief hospitalisation upon the psychiatric patient's household. *Acta Psychiatrica Scandinavica* 64:199-216.

23 Keogh, F. and Daly, I. (1994) *Family Burden in Community Psychiatry.* Dublin: Health Research Board.

Further Reading

Aldridge, J. and Becker, S. (1993) *Children who care - inside the world of young carers.* Loughborough: Loughborough University.

Atkinson, S.M. (1986) *Schizophrenia at home: A guide to helping the family.* New York: New York University Press.

Barrowclough, C. and Tarrier, N. (1992) *Families of Schizophrenic patients: Cognitive Behavioural Interventions.* London: Chapman & Hall.

Gopfert,M.V., Webster, J. and Seeman, M.V. (eds) (1996) *Parental Psychiatric Disorder: Distressed Parents and their Families.* Cambridge:CUP.

Orford, J. (1987) *Coping with disorder in the family.* London: Croom Helm.

Shepherd, G., Murray, A. and Muijen, M. (1994) *The different views of users, carers and professionals.* London: Sainsbury Centre.

SSI (1995) *A Way Ahead for Carers. Priorities for Managers and Practitioners.* London: HMSO.

SSI (1995) *Caring Today. National Inspection of Local Authority Support to Carers.* London: HMSO.

SSI (Social Services Inspectorate) (1995) *Partners in Caring* - The fourth annual report of the Chief Inspector of Social Services. London: HMSO.

SSI (1995) *What next for Carers? Findings from an SSI project.* London: HMSO.

Twigg, J. and Atkin, K.(1994) *Carers perceived: policy and practice in informal care.* Buckingham: Open University Press.

MENTALLY ILL PARENTS AND THEIR CHILDREN

INTRODUCTION

Health and social services authorities have a range of duties which include the provision of services for both children and adults. However, services for children are provided and administered separately from those for adults. Children are the responsibility of distinctive professional specialisms: paediatrics, child and adolescent mental health, and childcare teams in social services departments.

It is known that children who have a mentally ill parent are at a greater risk of developing problems in their own right than those whose parents are well. Yet children with a parent who is mentally ill may not attract services in their own right, unless they become conspicuously abused or neglected. Professionals involved with the care and support of adults with mental health difficulties may not be alert to the needs of children. They may be unfamiliar with how to obtain resources to support such children.

The result can be that the children of mentally ill parents fall through the net of professional concern. Children of lone parents are likely to be particularly vulnerable to living in situations where the quality of their care is badly affected.

CHILDREN'S NEEDS

The minimum needs of children are hard to specify; many children in the UK live in households that are poorly resourced in material or emotional terms. In assessing whether the needs of children are being met, the following areas should be considered:

- Does a parent (or adult in a parental role) generally anticipate the child's needs for food, clothing, sleep, play and safety?

- Does a parent respond to the child's initiatives, offer warm interactions, and respond to distress?

- Does a parent refer to the child positively, or describe them with warmth?

- Does a parent set reasonably age-appropriate boundaries to the child's behaviour?

- Does the parent expect to "look after" the child, rather than the child being expected to "look after" the parent?

- Does a parent offer a consistent and continuing relationship with the child, over time?

- Are any periods of separation managed reasonably in relation to the age of the child?

- As the child develops, is he or she supported in relationships with the world outside the immediate household?

- Is the child free from abuse?

The first two areas, anticipation of the child's needs and responding to the child, have been identified as crucial in the development of a positive attachment.[1] The child under about 3 years of age is particularly at risk of longer-term emotional difficulties if attachment needs are consistently neglected. A failure to develop a secure attachment in the very early years can lead to serious difficulties in personality development, affecting the capacity to make close relationships into adulthood. However, if the absence of a secure attachment within these early years is both identified and rectified a positive outcome is to be expected.

Children growing up in environments which offer them low levels of warmth, coupled with high levels of criticism, are also at risk of longer-term emotional and behavioural difficulty.[2]

MODULE 6

Lax or inconsistent boundaries on behaviour can be associated with impulsive physical abuse by parents. This "parenting style" essentially passive and with erratic discipline, was found to be associated with emotional unresponsiveness in parents and disturbed behaviour in children in one study.[3]

Activity

Think of a child or teenager in a family known to you personally (for example, a neighbour, friends, relatives) where you think the parenting is of a reasonably good standard.

- What does the parent do in response to the needs and challenges presented by the child?
- Identify the parenting behaviour and involvement with the child.
- What problems might a parent with a mental health problem have in parenting a similar child?

MENTAL HEALTH DIFFICULTIES IN PARENTS

Parenting brings its own stresses, particularly if the main carer of children lacks certain crucial supports. A number of studies have shown that women with young children are more likely to experience depression[4,5], although the relationship is mediated by other factors such as the quality of adult relationships available to the mother, economic resources, access to work opportunities and the mother's own parenting history.

Significant numbers of parents, mainly mothers, can therefore be expected to experience depression when children are young. Services need to attend to the likely impact upon children, and to offer appropriate support to children as well as parents.

Depression in adults can result in loss of energy or the ability to experience pleasure. Thinking may become negative and day to day activities may seem to lack meaning. There may be periods of intense self-preoccupation, or weeping and irrational anger.

Children looked after by a depressed parent may experience few expressions of positive warmth from the parent, and may become subject to criticism and blame. Their daily needs may be neglected by a parent who is listless and preoccupied. At times they may be called upon to comfort a parent who is in despair, or threatening suicide. If this situation persists, it is likely to erode the child's self-esteem, or create an overwhelming sense of anxiety and responsibility for the parent.

For younger children, failure to provide physical care and nurture, and warm responsiveness might result from parental depression. Older children may lack or lose positive interaction and stimulation, support in school and other outside activities, and appropriate discipline. All of these can have a cumulative impact on the child's development.

Depression is the most common mental health problem likely to be encountered amongst parents of dependent children. However, mental health professionals as well as those in children's services will also encounter adults with severe (psychotic) illnesses, such as schizophrenia or affective psychosis, who are parents of children. In the US it has been estimated that women with severe mental illness are almost as likely as other women to become mothers.[6] Sometimes the impairments resulting from their illness are so severe that these women are unable to look after their children. Either they are looked after by other family members, or they enter the public care system.

Mental health professionals need to be aware of the likely impact of severe mental illness on the ability to parent. Parents who have a psychotic illness have been described as making a "disorganised" contribution to the early attachment relationship with their children:

"When a parent's mind is filled with delusions, preoccupations or fears and her interpretation of events is dominated by abnormal beliefs, the capacity for necessary preoccupation with and sensitive perception of the children may be eliminated.

Elements of attachment that are observable .....may simply be missing, especially at the height of the psychotic episode. Attributions of intent and meaning of a child's actions may be so dominated by psychotic thinking, that the function of parenthood is completely undermined." [7]

The parent with active symptoms of, for example, schizophrenia, will have periods when his or her behaviour and communication are frightening, and unconnected to the needs of the child. The child's own ability to judge reality may be affected - children rely on their parents' perceptions of the world to develop their own understandings. A child whose parent holds paranoid delusional beliefs about the outside world may also experience the world as a frightening and hostile place.

Periods of unpredictable behaviour, and sudden separations when a parent is hospitalised will also have an impact upon the child. The management of these situations will crucially affect the child's experience of continuity and security, and may also contribute to problems of attachment.

In addition, a parent with psychotic symptoms may neglect or fail to protect a child, and in a minority of cases may actually abuse his or her child. We return later to the implications of this for service providers.

In reviewing the evidence of the impact of parental mental disorder on children, one author concludes that these children have themselves a "substantially increased risk" of psychiatric disorder.[8] Mentally ill parents are more likely than other parents to be lone parents, or the partners of other adults with psychiatric problems. This compounds the vulnerability of the child; if a child lives with two parents one of whom is not mentally ill, the diagnosis of the ill parent does not increase the risk of disturbance in the children.

Mental health professionals may also encounter adults who misuse drugs and alcohol, and who are also parenting young children. In some cases this will be a factor in marital or parental violence. Families where there is drug or alcohol misuse are likely to experience higher levels of financial problems and relationship difficulties, and there may also be police and criminal justice involvement. Four main areas of likely impact on children have been identified[9]:

- anti-social behaviour problems in children;

- school and learning problems;

- emotional problems;

- adolescence - likely to be more socially isolated, and have problems in making long-term close relationships.

Whilst not all children of parents who misuse alcohol or drugs will experience these problems, there will be higher levels of risk in families where there is also marital conflict, separation or divorce, violence, or inconsistent or ambivalent parenting.

PROTECTIVE AND RISK FACTORS

The impact of parental mental illness or alcohol or drug misuse upon children will be mediated by a range of other factors. These include:

- the child's access to the other parent and the mental well-being of the other parent;

- the child's age and stage of development when mental illness is first evident in a parent - the older the child, the less vulnerable to severe impact;

- the child's individual temperament and resilience;

- the severity, frequency and duration of episodes of mental illness in the parent;

- the degree of impairment to parenting functioning in the parent;

- the "style" of parenting in the family prior to mental health difficulties in the parent - indifferent or neglectful parenting can render a child particularly vulnerable;

- the wider social support available to the child from extended family, friends, teachers, or other adults;

- the resources available to the family to enable them to obtain other supports for the child (for example, activities);

- the level of disruption and separation experienced by the child, for any reason. Children precipitately admitted to care in their early years are more likely to experience longer-term attachment difficulties.

Severity of parental illness is not in itself the determining factor in assessing the impact upon a child. Professionals working in mental health services for adults will be familiar with using frameworks in which severity of illness is a key factor in priority for service (for example, the Care Programme Approach). Children need to be assessed by different criteria, as the cases below illustrate.

CASE STUDY: Debbie

Debbie (35 years) has two children aged 13 and 11 years. She is married to Dave (36 years) who is an education administrator.

Debbie has just experienced a first episode of manic depressive psychosis for which she was hospitalised under the Mental Health Act, 1983, for 3 weeks. Her mother and sister managed the care of the children whilst she was in hospital. Dave visited their schools and explained the situation, and this has been handled sensitively by teachers.

Debbie has recovered and takes regular medication. However, the condition is known to be likely to relapse.

The children were distressed by the change in their mother. However, they received explanation and support from Dave and their aunt.

CASE STUDY: Shelley

Shelley (25 years) is the lone parent of two children aged 4 years and 18 months. She is being treated by her GP for depression. Shelley finds it hard to respond to the demands of the children who she finds fretful. She often shouts and smacks the 4-year old, especially when she is tired and feeling low.

Shelley is on Income Support, and as she smokes there is little money left to do anything other than survive. She lives on a poor Council estate. Her sister also lives on the estate, but does not help, as Shelley has borrowed money from her and failed to repay it.

The children's father is now out of contact. The children have been in care (fostered) once during a previous family crisis. Shelley often talks about "putting them in care" for a break.

A number of points are evident from these two cases:

- Although Debbie has a mental illness which is described as "severe", the children are less at risk in many ways than those of Shelley;

- The experience of children is determined as much by family and social support, as by actual diagnosis;

- In terms of mental health services for adults, Debbie may receive more specialised attention and higher priority due to the severity of her illness;

- Children need a separate child-focused assessment of their needs, and services in their own right.

INTERVENTION WITH MENTALLY ILL PARENTS AND THEIR CHILDREN

Assessment of the needs of adults with mental health problems should include an assessment of any children they are looking after. This is of particular importance when the adult is a lone parent, or the main carer of children.

In some cases there will be a clear conflict of interest between the needs of the parent and those of the children. The parenting performance may be insufficient to meet the minimal needs of the children, even with support. Yet the role of parent may be highly valued by the person who is mentally ill. In these cases there are difficult decisions to be faced by professionals.

In many cases the parent will be able to offer some parenting functions, or will be able to parent adequately between episodes of illness. Support services should be tailored to address the needs of dependent children which are not met by the parent, in addition to supporting the parent him or herself. A number of innovative projects such as Newpin (Peckham, London) and Home Start (Nottingham) aim to support vulnerable parents and children.[10]

If the minimal needs of the children cannot be met, even with the support of available services, alternative care plans for the children may need to be considered. In a small number of cases, statutory intervention under *The Children Act, 1989* may be necessary (see Module 3). The care of dependent children must not be allowed to fall below an acceptable standard in the perceived interests of the mentally ill parent.

COMMUNICATING WITH CHILDREN WHOSE PARENT HAS A MENTAL HEALTH PROBLEM

It is important not to overlook the need to talk to older children about their parent's mental health problems. In some families, the other parent or a relative will be able to do this. Some parents will be able to explain their own mental health difficulties to their children. In other circumstances, child care or mental health professionals may be in the best position to help the child make sense of the experience. Normally this would be with the agreement of the parents.

For young children, the most urgent task is to ensure that the child's own needs are met. Simple explanation about the parent's absence or changed behaviour should be given, taking account of the child's level of understanding.

Older children must also have their needs addressed, but may even so experience thoughts and feelings about their parent's condition which might be helped by discussion, explanation and reassurance. These might include:

- anxiety that they are "to blame";

- anger and blame towards the ill parent;

- anger and blame towards others (for example, an absent parent);

- anxiety that they too will become mentally ill;

- social embarrassment and fear of stigma;

- fear of the ill parent;

- anxiety about younger siblings;

- fear of having no-one to look after them;

- grief about the loss of the relationship with the ill parent.

Not all children will be able to use "talking help". Some children are able to express their thoughts and feelings directly. In other cases feelings are expressed as "difficult behaviour". This can include:

- resistance to talking about the illness or the ill parent;

- acting as if nothing has happened;

- anger and rejection towards the ill parent; refusing to see them;

- problematic behaviour within or outside the home.

These children should not be regarded as either resilient or unfeeling. "Difficult" behaviour is commonly a sign that children are having difficulty coping with their experiences. They need support, and may be able to talk through their feelings at a later stage.

A wide range of other behaviours may be exhibited by children experiencing the stress of mental illness. Some may need skilled therapeutic help via child and adolescent mental health services.

THE CHILDREN ACT, 1989

The provisions of *The Children Act, 1989* are summarised in Module 3 "Legislation and Policy". The Act incorporates a number of key principles which are helpful in considering both needs and risks in relation to the children of parents with a mental illness.

The principle that the child's welfare is paramount establishes that, even where parents are vulnerable or coping with circumstances not of their own making, in a conflict of interests the child's welfare must always be the paramount consideration.

Services can be provided under *The Children Act, 1989*, if the child is defined as a "child in need" in the terms of the Act. Section 17 of *The Children Act, 1989*, states that a child is "in need" if:

- " he is unlikely to achieve or maintain, or to have the opportunity of achieving or maintaining, a reasonable standard of health or development without the provision for him of services by a local authority....;

- his health or development is likely to be significantly impaired, or further impaired, without the provision for him of such services; or

- he is disabled." (section 17(1))

A further principle of the Act is that services must be provided in such a way as to promote the upbringing of children by their families provided that is consistent with the child's welfare.

Within these provisions, services could be provided to children whose parents have a mental illness. Services can include nursery or day care, family centres and holiday activities for children.

The Children Act, 1989, also provides the framework for the protection of children at risk. Care or Supervision Orders can be made by the Courts in respect of children experiencing "significant harm" (or likely significant harm) due to the standard of care provided. Significant harm includes both ill treatment and impairment of the child's health or

development. A further principle of the Act is that no Court order will be made if the protection of the child can be achieved without an order.

The assessment and decision-making process in child protection is detailed in guidance.[11] This includes multi-disciplinary involvement, the arena for which is the child protection conference. In cases involving mentally ill parents, professionals from the adult mental health services should be part of this process.

In a recent report into children killed by their parents, about a third of notified cases in one year were clearly identified as involving a psychiatrically ill parent. One of the main findings of the report was the lack of integration of children's services and adult mental health services in working with the families, the majority of whom were known to either or both services. In 78% of the cases there were existing child protection issues at the point of the death. Most of the perpetrators had a history of admission to psychiatric units, and the majority had a history of known violence.[12]

In extreme and rare cases, even with the provision of support services, children with a parent who is mentally ill can be judged to have reached the threshold for "significant harm". They can then be removed from the care of the parents. However, the Act establishes the principle that contact with parents continues unless there is specific reason to forbid this.

Professionals working with adults who are mentally ill should be aware of the provisions of *The Children Act, 1989*, in relation to both children in need and children at risk. The Act provides a framework for intervention which is specifically child-focused.

THE CARERS (RECOGNITION AND SERVICES) ACT, 1995

Under this Act, young people who provide care for their parents are entitled to an assessment of their needs. Any services to children and young people following such an assessment will be provided under *The Children Act, 1989 - The Carers (Recognition and Services) Act, 1995,* does not confer an entitlement to services.

The Carers (Recognition and Services) Act, 1995, aimed to ensure that the needs of carers were taken account of in assessments of adults. The guidance to the Act emphasises that when assessing a young carer, the needs of the child and the parenting role of the adult must be considered.

SERVICES

Adults with mental health problems are assessed and receive services via the twin frameworks of *The NHS and Community Care Act, 1990* and the Care Programme Approach, 1990. These frameworks are appropriate to the needs of adults, but do not specifically address the needs of children.

Ideally services should support both adults and children in families under stress because of adult mental health difficulties. The administrative separation of services for adults and children should not mean that children's needs are neglected, or seen as secondary to those of the ill adult.

• •

DILEMMA: Mr Willis (41 years) & Darren (13 years)

Mr. Willis's wife left him for a new partner 8 years ago. She took their daughter but left Darren with his father. There is now no contact and it is not known where she lives.

Mr. Willis worked as a factory supervisor. He was made redundant 6 years ago and has not worked since. He is a solitary man who has no social contact and is unfriendly to neighbours.

The family GP is alerted by the school nurse that Darren has been found to have untreated scabies, and seems neglected and withdrawn. He has many absences from school, but has not triggered any substantial concern.

Mr. Willis responds to a request to bring Darren to the surgery. Mr. Willis is hostile and suspicious when asked about how he manages. However, the GP has known the family for a number of years. He is a fund-holder with CPN support at the surgery. He persuades Mr. Willis to allow a CPN to visit "to see if he can help in any way."

The CPN is shocked by the state of the house. Darren sleeps on a couch downstairs with only an old blanket. Food and dirty clothes are trampled on the floor. He feels that Mr. Willis may be depressed, but he is also rejecting of any help, such as a home help.

The CPN alerts the children's section of the Social Services Department. He expresses the view that there are no grounds for compulsory intervention in respect of Mr. Willis, but that perhaps Darren would be "better off in Care".

What issues might be considered?

There is no obvious solution to a situation like this. Despite the squalor of the home, Mr. Willis may have given Darren a stability which the public care system would be unlikely to replicate. The following are suggestions for the direction of work with the family:

• Every attempt should be made to build a relationship with Mr. Willis and Darren on a voluntary basis;

• The GP (or CPN) may be able to emphasise the concerns about Darren, and persuade Mr. Willis to accept some help;

• An assessment of Darren's needs and Mr. Willis's parenting needs to be made;

• It needs to be established whether Mr. Willis has a mental health problem, whether this can be treated, and how it affects his parenting;

• Services should support both Mr. Willis and Darren;

• Services should work together flexibly, enabling Mr. Willis to get a range of help from the source most acceptable to him.

What other issues might be considered?

• •

Professionals working in services for adults may not be aware of the range of services that may be available to support children. The following is a summary of commonly available services.

- Health visitors and community midwives: visit mothers of young children at home and are skilled in the monitoring of early health and development.

- School nurses: broad health screening of school-age children at intervals. Immunisation. School nurse in larger schools available to respond to health-related issues.

- General Practitioners: will have a long-term knowledge of the health of the family. May contribute a family perspective to assessment.

- Child and Adolescent Mental Health Services: specialist assessment and treatment of child mental health difficulties. Out-patient care; some in-patient units.

- Schools: will have knowledge of children based on continuing contact in a group setting. Primary school class teachers and secondary school class tutors are generally the best contact in respect of the individual child, being in a position to monitor educational and social development.

- Nurseries and family centres: in a position to support and monitor the under-fives.

- Social services departments: have a range of services and staff; offer family support, day services and residential services for children. Responsible for placing children with foster carers. Offer services to children in need, children in need of protection, young offenders and those leaving care. Social services departments act as both purchasers and providers of children's services. They also purchase services from voluntary and independent providers.

Professionals in the field of adult mental health need to work closely with these services if they are to deliver effective family interventions that take account of the needs of children. This should involve child care social workers being involved in meetings concerning the mental health problems of parents, wherever parenting is an issue of concern.

References

1   Bowlby J. (1969) *Attachment and Loss. Vol.1 Attachment.* London: Hogarth Press.

2   Department of Health (1995) *Child Protection: Messages from the Research. Studies in Child Protection.* London: HMSO.

3   Waterhouse L., Pitcairn T., McGhee J., Secker J. and'Sullivan C. (1993) 'Evaluating parenting in child physical abuse' in Waterhouse L. *Child Abuse and Child Abusers.* London: Jessica Kingsley.

4   Brown G. and Harris T. (1978) *Social Origins of Depression.* London: Tavistock.

5   Paykel E. (1991) 'Depression in Women'. *British Journal of Psychiatry*, 158, (suppl.10), 22-29.

6   Mowbray C.T., Oyserman D., Zemencuk J.K. and Ross S.R. (1995) 'Motherhood for women with serious mental illness: pregnancy, childbirth and the postpartum period. *American Journal of Orthopsychiatry*, 65, (1), 21-38.

7   Hill J. (1996) 'Parental psychiatric disorder and the attachment relationship' (page 12) in Gopfert M., Webster J. and Seeman M.V.(eds) *Parental Psychiatric Disorder: distressed parents and their families.* Cambridge: Cambridge University Press.

8   Hall A. (1996) 'Parental psychiatric disorder and the developing child' in Gopfert M, Webster J and Seeman M.V.(eds) *Parental Psychiatric Disorder: distressed parents and their families.* Cambridge: Cambridge University Press.

9   Velleman R. (1996) 'Alcohol and drug problems in parents: an overview of the impact on children and the implications for practice' in Gopfet M., Webster J. and Seeman M.V. (eds) *Parental Psychiatric Disorder: distressed parents and their families.* Cambridge: Cambridge University Press.

10 Sayce L. and Sherlock J. (1994) *'Good practices in services for women with child-related needs' in Women and Mental Health: An information pack of mental health services for women in the United Kingdom.* London: Good Practices in Mental Health.

11 Home Office/Department of Health/Department of Education and Science/Welsh Office (1991) *Working Together under the Children Act 1989: a guide to arrangements for inter- agency cooperation for the protection of children from abuse.* London: HMSO.

12 Falkov A. (1996) *Study of Working Together "Part 8" Reports: Fatal Child Abuse and Parental Psychiatric Disorder. An analysis of 100 Area Child Protection Committee case reviews conducted under the terms of Part 8 of Working Together under the Children Act, 1989.* London: Department of Health.

● ●

This module - "Users, Carers and Children of Parents with Mental Health Problems" - is one of 7 modules in "Learning Materials on Mental Health - An Introduction" . The other modules include:

Module 1 - "Recognition of Mental Health Problems"
Module 2 - "Intervention and Management"
Module 3 - "Legislation and Guidance"
Module 4 - "Special Client Groups"
Module 5 - "Special Issues"
Module 7 - "Sample Training Exercises"

A sister set of materials is also available for professionals involved in assessing risk - "Learning Materials on Mental Health Risk Assessment"

module 7

TRAINER'S EXERCISES

....

AIMS & OBJECTIVES

After you have used/considered the exercises in this module
you should be better able to:

- Identify your own and other perspectives and
  assumptions on "mental health" and "mental illness".

- Discuss ways of problem-solving, intervening and
  managing mental health situations.

- Describe the skills, roles and responsibilities of
  different workers within a multi- disciplinary approach.

- Discuss the key themes and issues arising from
  recent legislation and guidance.

- Evaluate the extent to which the needs and views of
  users and carers are involved in the development of
  mental health services.

INTRODUCTION TO THIS SAMPLE OF TRAINING EXERCISES

There are 12 exercises.

All have been designed for a group workshop setting but several are open to being tackled by an individual worker engaged in private study. Whichever way they are used **interaction with others** is seen as beneficial in terms of generating an exchange of perceptions, information and skills and potentially some reframing of individual assumptions and approaches. A group workshop membership of 12-16 is proposed as the most fruitful for both trainer(s) and participants. One of the group leaders should be an experienced mental health social worker.

Each exercise has been linked to one or more modules. This may be, or feel like, an artificial division as a number clearly span the boundaries and content of different modules. All, for example, can be linked to Modules 4 and 5, covering special client groups and issues in mental health care. Different exercises will reveal or suggest different linkages to different people. Trainers, workshop participants and those engaged in private study are, therefore, invited to use the exercises as they feel they might assist learning, bearing in mind the stated purpose and any notes of guidance.

Each exercise has a common structure, hopefully to render them accessible and easy to use.

Three final points, which in other contexts might be described as a "health warning":

1) It is now common practice to establish "ground rules" for behaviour in training workshops. These exercises assume that this work will have been done to enable participants and trainers to work together in a spirit of partnership and confidence, whilst recognising the qualities of difference.

2) Many of the exercises are capable of triggering feelings, personal experiences and views which may prove unsettling for individuals and the workshop as a whole. These dynamics need to be recognised and managed constructively. Careful preparation, facilitation and debriefing cannot be emphasised enough.

3) Trainers should bear in mind that the strengths of people with mental health problems should be "drawn out" in discussion, so that participants are not left with a solely negative image of mental illness.

We hope that you will have fun in the pursuit of serious learning.

EXERCISE CONTENTS

1. **Perspectives on Mental Health**

2. **Mental Health and Stigma**

3. **Assumptions and Stereotypes**

4. **Roles and Responsibilities**

5. **What would you say?**

6. **Service Planning**

7. **What is the problem?**

8. **The Quiz**

9. **Personal Audit: What do you know?**

10. **On the Receiving End**

11. **Involving Consumers**

12. **What if.........? A Guided Fantasy**

MODULE 7

| Module One | **Recognition of Mental Health Problems** |

Potential Training Exercise: Perspectives on Mental Health

PURPOSE/OBJECTIVES

To highlight the different perspectives on "mental health" and "mental illness".

MATERIALS

1. Flip chart and pens.
2. Group instruction cards (see overleaf).

Time for exercise: 30 - 45 minutes

PROCESS

1. The trainer presents the notion of a debate in which the workshop participants are invited to discuss some of the key perspectives, according to a given role.

2. The motion for the debate is:

   "This House believes that depression is a stress response to difficult circumstances." [This motion can be written on flip chart or given out on prepared sheets.]

3. The participants are invited to divide into at least four different perspective groups, self-selecting from the following possibilities:

   *   Psychiatrists
   *   Social Workers, Social Care Managers
   *   Patients/Users
   *   Carers
   *   GPs
   *   CPNs

   The number of groups will depend upon the size of the workshop. 3 - 4 members per group is a suggested minimum.

4. Each group meets to consider the above motion for 10 - 15 minutes.

5. During the group discussions, the trainer circulates and verifies which groups will be arguing for and against the motion.

6. After the agreed time has elapsed, the groups return to a plenary where the debate takes place, with the trainer(s) acting as Chair for the proceedings. The participants are encouraged to assert their perspective in the spirit of debate and to enjoy the exercise.

NOTES FOR TRAINERS AND PARTICIPANTS

1. This exercise works best if participants can be encouraged to view it as part serious, part fun, by entering into the spirit of debate, perhaps even taking a position they would not wholly endorse in practice in order to highlight differences and the implications.

2. All "live" exercises of this kind are capable of triggering strongly held views and personal experiences. This can be a powerful dynamic which will need monitoring.

3. Variation: Depending upon the size of the workshop, you may wish to identify observers/assessors whose task would be to feed back their perceptions of the quality of the arguments presented and the one which they see as the most persuasive.

4. Trainer(s) may wish to prepare their own "prompt cards" identifying likely differences/ controversial areas/ dilemmas, for example, effectiveness of treatment, cultural perspectives, and so on... These can be used, if necessary, to add material if the debate is "flat" and/or to draw things to a close.

| Module Two | Intervention (Service Settings) |

Potential Training Exercise: Service Planning

PURPOSE/OBJECTIVES

To familiarise group members with some service planning issues, when addressing the mental health needs of a given population.

MATERIALS

- Task sheets (overleaf)
- Flip chart and pens

PROCESS

The students should work in four small groups.

Each group is presented with an instruction card (overleaf).

Each small group should work on one of the following tasks:

1. Draw plans for the building itself.
2. Draw up a programme for a week for those wishing to attend the centre.
3. Design an information/publicity leaflet for service users and professionals.
4. Write a job description for a "front-line" member of staff.

Feedback in full group discussion.

NOTES FOR TRAINER

The plans for the building should trigger discussion about the range of activities, the need for private and small group areas, and communal areas. Is there planning for the potential needs of women, and cultural needs (for example, a prayer room)? How is staff space addressed?

Activities - Is there a balance between "joining in" and "opting out"? How are activities decided? Can users initiate new activities?

Leaflet - Highlight
1) things of importance to users - ease of access, friendliness, coffee/lunch and so on,
2) The importance of simple language,
3) The availability in different languages.

Staff - Areas of discussion are likely to include a range of skills, attitudes and equal opportunities issues.

TIME

About an hour with at least 20 minutes for the small group activity.

GROUP INSTRUCTION SHEET

Your district has a population of 260,000 and is a town within a county administration. The 1991 Census indicates that the adult population of the town consists of the following ethnic groups :

88.5%	White European
8.0%	Pakistani
1.5%	Bengali
1.0%	African-Caribbean
1.0%	Other ethnic groups

The town has high levels of unemployment, and traditional industries are in decline.

A new mental health day centre is to be built in the town, offering a service primarily to those with severe and longer-term mental illnesses. The aim is to support people in living in the community. The facility will offer two main kinds of support:

(1) support in participating in "mainstream" activities;

(2) support within the facility for those who prefer to remain there during the day.

Module Two/Four	Intervention and Management Special Client Groups - Mental Health

Potential Training Exercise: "What is the problem?"

PURPOSE/OBJECTIVE

To invite participants to employ a systematic problem solving approach as a means of developing good practice in mental health.

MATERIALS

1. Selection of case studies - see below.
2. Flip chart and pens.
3. A copy of the key questions for the group to address (see overleaf).

PROCESS

1. The trainer presents the model of the "Problem Solving Tree" and/or gives brief input on problem solving processes, with a handout. (See overleaf)

2. The workshop participants form small groups (4 - 6 members), each participant having a copy of a selected case study - (see overleaf).

3. The groups are invited to work at key questions (overleaf) and record the outcomes on a flip chart.

4. The groups give brief feedback on outcome with discussion.

PROBLEM SOLVING INPUT

There is a lot written about effective problem solving (for example, De Bono). Critical elements are said to be:

- Make sure you're working at the right problem, rather than the symptoms.
- Look carefully at the roots or causes in seeking **to define which problem** you want/need to tackle.
- Generate a range of possible solutions - from the realistic to the ideal.
- Identify the consequences or implications of each solution.
- Evaluate the positive/negative/most likely way forward.
- Monitor and review.

The problem solving tree offers a graphic structure or process for putting this into effect. Most situations faced by social services and health care professionals are multi-faceted and interventions may often be service rather than needs led. Identifying the "right" problem(s) may be more cost effective.

NOTES FOR TRAINERS AND PARTICIPANTS

1. This exercise can be kept brief or extended as necessary. One variation, therefore, is to focus mainly on the issue of defining the problem without pursuing any solutions.

2. A range of studies are suggested overleaf but you may have other case studies with which you are more familiar, or which relate particularly to the practice interests of workshop members.

3. Sometimes case studies are found wanting because there may be other pieces of information that participants feel they need. Cautious licence can be given in these circumstances to imagine or invent a "missing piece", drawing upon practice experience.

4. Different groups may well identify different problems within the same case study. This can be a critical discussion point and illustrates the importance of defining the problem.

PROBLEM SOLVING INPUT

- Make sure you're working at the right problem, rather than the symptoms.

- Look carefully at the roots or causes in seeking **to define which problem** you want/need to tackle.

- Generate a range of possible solutions - from the realistic to the ideal.

- Identify the consequences or implications of each solution.

- Evaluate the positive/negative/most likely way forward.

- Monitor and review.

KEY QUESTIONS FOR THE GROUP IN ADDRESSING A CASE STUDY

- What is the problem? What are the roots/causes? Who is the client?

- What alternative solutions/strategies might be generated?

- What would be the consequences of these - positive/negative?

- Which solution/strategy would the group employ?

- Record and be prepared to feed back to the main group.

SELECTION OF CASE STUDIES [FIVE]

Case Study One: The Stapletons

A 'phone call is received from Mrs Stapleton who is expressing considerable concern about the well-being of her grandson, Paul. At present Paul is living with his mother, Josephine, Mrs Stapleton's youngest daughter. Josephine is also known as Jo. This is the family background according to Mrs Stapleton........

Jo is separated from her husband, Terry, who left the marital home three months ago. They had been partners for six years - Paul is 4 years old and their only child. Jo has a daughter, Lisa, now 11 years old, from a previous marriage. Lisa lives with her father and his second wife but visits her mother and half brother almost daily as the two families live on the same estate.

Jo has a history of mental health difficulties dating from Lisa's birth after which she was diagnosed as having puerperal depression. Jo was very anxious about her baby and was mistakenly convinced that Lisa had Downes Syndrome. Jo eventually spent three months in a psychiatric hospital undergoing a variety of therapies/treatments, including ECT and group discussion with other patients considered to be chronically depressed.

Since that original episode Jo has apparently been "well" for most of the time, although from time to time she has experienced extreme reactions to stress and delusions that her husband was having an affair with a number of their friends and relatives. Further hospitalisation has been suggested at times by the Consultant undertaking domiciliary visits but this has been resisted.

Jo is a rather unassertive woman, very gentle and kind and according to her mother very easily led and exploited. A year ago Jo became involved with a devout religious sect and in particular with the leader, Stefan. Jo is now apparently having visions of Christ, is expressing deep contentment. She tells her mother that she feels fulfilled. All Jo's family and friends believe that she is hallucinating and has become ill again, although Paul is apparently well cared for and there are no signs of abuse or neglect. Mrs Stapleton is, however, concerned about the effect that Jo's "illness" is having upon

Paul, who seems increasingly withdrawn and clings to his grandmother and to his sister, Lisa, when they leave after family visits. Mrs Stapleton, in her seventies, lives in a different part of the City, is caring for a husband with health problems and feels that something should be done soon. She has clearly played a dominant role in Jo's life and is threatened by the degree of control that Stefan is enjoying over her daughter.

Case Study Two: Janet and Liam

Janet, a white woman of 49 years, has been married to Liam for twenty-five years. Six months ago he was forced to take redundancy ("early retirement") at 54 years. Always a fairly heavy drinker, Liam is now increasingly dependent upon alcohol to cope with everyday stress and also the pain of an arthritic spine. When he has been drinking, he becomes abusive - particularly towards Janet. Liam accuses her of infidelity and rails endlessly and bitterly about the firm/department/company he used to work for. He feels abused after giving long service and that his back problems stemmed from his working life.

Liam has few friends, has always in the past been close to Janet but seems to her "like two people." He is particularly aggressive and abusive towards his adult children when they visit, seeking argument and confrontation over trivial matters and turning political discussion into personal conflict. Janet is now at the end of her tether. She loves her husband dearly and, when he is sober or trying to stop drinking, she is moved to tenderness and forgiveness by his shame and remorse. However, when he's been drinking, she feels powerless to combat the lies (hiding bottles, spending excessively and so on) as well as his threats.

The G.P. is a family friend and Janet is wary of involving her. Liam refuses to seek help and puts on a facade of being "OK!" towards everyone outside the family.

Case Study Three: Mary and Arthur

Mary is married to Arthur. They are both white, of
Lithuanian/Jewish origin, and in their early seventies. Arthur
is admitted to hospital following a heart attack . Whilst on the
acute medical ward, it becomes apparent that Arthur is very
confused, and he tends to wander restlessly at night. Signs
of acute infection are investigated, but finally he is diagnosed
as having Alzheimer's Disease.

Mary has been struggling to cope without assistance as
Arthur's mental difficulties have increased over the past two
years. Despite some encouragement and support from their
son and his wife, Mary has been reluctant to admit that there
is a problem, in part because Arthur is very hard of hearing.
Arthur repeats the same phrase over and over, disturbs her
sleep, pulls out the catheter he now requires for urinary
incontinence and changes the television and radio
programmes over at 2-3 minute intervals in frustration.
Mary had thought that things would improve if he had the
right kind of help with his hearing, but seems relieved now
that help is being offered.

Case Study Four: Alan

Alan is African-Caribbean, 15 years old and until recently was
a lively lad, enjoying school; performing in school
shows/plays, in the football team and doing reasonably well
in tests/exams. He is bright enough to stay on at school after
his GCSE's which are coming up in a few months' time. The
school is now concerned as Alan seems withdrawn, listless
and often very tired in class - frequently failing to complete
homework. This is unusual but most attempts to talk to him
have met with little success and problems at home have been
suspected for a while. Alan has now confided in the football
coach that his mother is finding it harder and harder to go out
of the house, is nervous of strangers calling and is
increasingly leaving the care of the two youngest children and
the running of the household to Alan. Alan's father is a long-
distance lorry driver, who is rarely home. He and his father
do not get on well - Alan it seems blames his mother's state
of mental health on his father's job and preferred lifestyle.

Case Study Five: Karen

Karen is white, 26 years old and discloses at work that she
had been sexually abused as a teenager. She is wondering if
she is likely to abuse her own children because of this. She is
encouraged to refer herself by a colleague.

Karen was abused by her grandfather from age 11-16 years
and recently discovered that he also abused her mother and
her sister in the past. The whole family still meet regularly and
the sexual abuse is buried beneath an "OK!" facade. Everyone
seems to be in denial. Karen's grandmother died earlier this
year.

Karen has ambivalent feelings in all her relationships. It
emerges that she is self-harming: cutting her legs and arms
with a Stanley knife when she feels desperate and frequently
taking small overdoses with pills and alcohol. She has a
boyfriend, Clive, who wants them to marry - he is unaware of
her drug and alcohol abuse and "cutting". They do not have
an open sexual relationship, for example, they do not undress
in front of each other and, although they have had intercourse
a few times, this produces a "frozenness" in Karen and
flashbacks to her grandfather's abuse.

Karen presents as wary and erratic, alternately talkative and
silent for minutes on end. She says that cutting herself at
least shows she is "alive" - that the blood flow demonstrates
this. She is unsure whether to marry Clive and is fearful of
having her own children. Sometimes she says she becomes
violently angry and lashes out at her boyfriend/mother or
whoever gets in the way - at other times she becomes
distressed.

Karen refuses to seek medical help.

Module Three | Legislation and Guidance

Potential Training Exercise: 'The Quiz'

PURPOSE/OBJECTIVE

To reinforce and extend learning about facts, intent and implications arising within different elements of mental health legislation and guidance.

MATERIALS

1. Copies of 'The Quiz' (overleaf).
2. The answers (overleaf).
3. A small prize.

PROCESS

1. Consider the timing of this exercise - a beginning warm-up? or post session monitoring activity? or end of course refresher, and so on.... (or morning after overnight "homework").

2. *Either*
   a) Distribute copies of the questionnaire to each participant, or to a pair/trio, and set a time limit for completion, **or**
   b) Read the questions aloud and invite participants to record their own answers.

3. When completed, ask participants to exchange their answer sheets for marking.

4. Trainer reads the answers aloud, using opportunities as relevant to discuss any issues arising.

5. Award a small prize for the participant (group) with most points?! (26 is the top score possible)

NOTES FOR PARTICIPANTS AND TRAINERS

1. We suggest that this exercise is managed in a light way (good natured banter, groans, cheers and smiles will be a reflection of, and contribute to, group cohesion rather than a heavy sense of competition).

2. It would be helpful to have sources at hand including Module Three, copies of legislation, handouts to confirm any doubts expressed or to reinforce discussion points.

'The Quiz'

1. When was the Care Programme Approach introduced? (1 point)

2. When were Supervision Registers introduced and name two of the four specific purposes described in the Health Service Guidelines. (3 points)

3. What was the overall suicide rate per 100,000 population in 1990? (1 point)

4. Name the different periods of time for which individuals may be compulsorily admitted to hospital under The Mental Health Act, 1983 and the specific sections of the Act relating to these. (3 points)

5. What specific powers are given to those acting as Guardians under The Mental Health Act, 1983? (3 points)

6. Why has guardianship been only infrequently used to date? (2 points)

7. What key themes can you identify in service policy and provision in mental health in the 1990s? (4 points)

8. What percentage of the Mental Illness Specific Grant has to be contributed by the local social services department? (1 Point)

9. Identify the four types of risk which were specified in the Mental Health (Patients in the Community) Act, 1995. (4 Points)

10. Name at least four of the six key objectives of the White Paper Caring for People, 1989. (4 Points)

ANSWERS TO 'THE QUIZ'

1. April 1991.
2. 1994 (April)

Purposes:

- to provide a care plan that aims to reduce the risk and ensure that the patient's care needs are reviewed regularly and that contact by a key worker is maintained.
- to provide a point of contact for authorised health and social services staff to determine whether individuals under the Care Programme Approach are at risk.
- to plan for the facilities and resources necessary to meet the needs of this group of patients (i.e. those deemed to be high risk or capable of dangerous behaviour).
- to identify those patients who should receive the highest priority for care and active follow up.

3. 11.0 per 100,000 population.
4. (I)   Section 2 - 28 days maximum (for assessment)
   (ii) Section 3 - 6 months maximum (for treatment)
   (iii) Section 4 - 72 hours maximum (urgent necessity).
5. (I)   The power to require the individual to live in a specific place.
   (ii) The power to require the person to attend for medical treatment, occupation, education or training.
   (iii) The power to require access to the person by a doctor, social worker or any other person.
6. (I)   Guardianship is little used because it is seen as lacking in powers of enforcement.
   (ii) Also, concern about resource implications which will fall on local authorities if it is used frequently.
7. Some key themes:
   (I)   Efficient targeting of mental health services.
   (ii) Quality control in the delivery of health and social services.
   (iii) Effective multi-disciplinary intervention.
   (iv) Risk and dangerousness.
   N.B. Discretionary points could be awarded for alternative, credible responses.
8. 30 per cent.
9. (I)   Harm to the health of the patient.
   (ii) Harm to the safety of the patient.
   (iii) Harm to the safety of other persons.
   (iv) Harm arising from the patient being seriously exploited
10. (I)   To promote the development of domiciliary, day and respite services to enable people to live in their own homes whenever feasible and sensible
    (ii) To ensure that service providers make practical support for carers a high priority
    (iii) To make proper assessment of need and good care management the cornerstone of high quality care
    (iv) To promote the development of a flourishing independent sector alongside good quality public services.
    (v)   To clarify the responsibilities of agencies and make it easier to hold them to account for their performance
    (vi) To secure better value for taxpayers' money by introducing a new funding structure for social care.

Module Three	Legislation and Guidance

Potential Training Exercise: Personal Audit: 'What do I know?'

PURPOSE/OBJECTIVES

To identify and enhance working knowledge of the legislation and guidance about mental health provision.

MATERIALS

1. All participants will need paper and pen or equivalent.
2. Flip chart and pens.

PROCESS

1. All participants are invited to make their own notes about those elements of the Mental Health Legislation and guidance of which they feel they have a reasonable working knowledge,

   For example, I have a good working knowledge of.........
   "Section 3 of the *Mental Health Act, 1983*, I have seen it used quite often and my experience is..." or "the use of the Mental Illness Specific Grant 1991 - some of the positive uses and flaws, and so on."
   (10 minutes)

2. Trainer then invites participants to circulate and compare with others, possibly adding to their individual lists as comparisons trigger memory or add to the stock of working knowledge. (15 minutes)

3. The participants are invited to cluster into groups of four:

   • to exchange and compare their knowledge
   • to produce a graphic presentation of their composite knowledge, for example, a cartoon picture of their composite worker equipped with working knowledge.

4. The groups briefly present their graphics to the rest of the workshop.

NOTES FOR TRAINERS AND PARTICIPANTS

1. This can be one way of gaining a sense of the levels of experience/knowledge of the group members at any stage in a workshop process. It could, therefore, be a challenging warm-up, a monitoring tool or end of workshop review.

2. A spirit of exchange and development supported by an informal fun approach, certainly in the suggested graphics, is recommended to minimise any sense of competition or "heaviness" in this exercise.

Module Two/Six | **Intervention and Management**
Service Users and Carers

Potential Training Exercise: "On the receiving end"

PURPOSE/OBJECTIVES

- To consider personal/family networks available in the event of mental health difficulties.
- To identify expectations of professionals.
- To compare these perceptions with current provision and to highlight a user perspective.

MATERIALS

1. Flip chart and pens.
2. A copy of the scenario and questions (overleaf).
3. Sufficient room for participants to have quiet/private space for discussion and reflection.
3. Time for exercise: 45 minutes - 1 hour.

PROCESS

1. The trainer presents the exercise as one in which participants are invited to reflect on what it might be like if they were to receive a diagnosis of "mental illness" and what their expectations would be of the professionals involved, and their own personal networks.

2. The participants are invited to work in pairs with someone with whom they feel comfortable.

3. The trainer asks the pairs to discuss and make their own notes in response to a brief scenario and related questions (See overleaf).

4. Allow between 15 - 30 minutes for the pairs to consider these questions, to be followed by a plenary session in which the trainer facilitates feedback, recording the main points on a central flip chart.

NOTES FOR TRAINERS AND PARTICIPANTS

1. All "live" exercises of this nature are capable of triggering feelings or past experiences inside those involved. Any feelings of discomfort, criticism or oppression will need to be acknowledged sensitively and constructively. In a large group, trainers may wish to establish firm boundaries, to keep the sharing of personal experiences within manageable limits.

2. It is suggested that the plenary feedback session focuses on the skills/qualities expected and how this compares with the services that participants and others currently provide.

SCENARIO AND QUESTIONS

You have been feeling confused, unable to cope and have stress levels beyond your previous experience. On visiting your GP, you are told that you are suffering from some form of mental illness and given a prescription for one of the anxiolytic or hypnotic group of drugs, for example, diazepam or temazepam. She also suggests strongly that you should see a Psychiatrist.

NETWORKS:

* Who would you be able to draw upon for day to day care and support emotionally and practically?

* What are your networks, their strengths and limitations, particularly if your condition does not respond to treatment and becomes long term?

SKILLS/QUALITIES EXPECTED:

* What core skills, qualities, style of approach would you want the relevant professionals to display towards you? For example, technical knowledge, listening skills.

* Which of these would be your priority?

MODULE 7

Module Six — Services Users and Carers

Potential Training Exercise: Involving Consumers

PURPOSE/OBJECTIVES

To identify and explore the issues when seeking to involve service users and carers in service development. To enable exchange of experience and ideas. To enhance creativity.

MATERIALS

Flip chart and pens. Time for exercise: 1 hour 30 minutes.

PROCESS

1. The workshop participants are invited to form small groups (4 - 6 members) and to consider themselves as an agency team or a multi-disciplinary working group charged with designing policy and practice guidelines for ensuring effective service user and carer involvement in the proposed development of a drop-in centre for people with mental health problems.

2. Groups are strongly advised that there are no restrictions on what they create. They are positively encouraged to design what they would regard as the ideal plan.

3. Group activity [1 hour].

4. Each group presents findings in as imaginative a way as possible.

NOTES FOR TRAINERS AND PARTICIPANTS

1. There may well be participants who bring personal experience of such developments. This should be acknowledged but exchange of ideas and assumptions in an open and questioning way is preferable to the dominance of alleged expertise.

2. Some participants may challenge the notion of designing an ideal plan as unhelpful in a climate of restricted resources and political agendas. Part of this exercise is about creativity and fun. Equally, it may be pertinent in the final plenary to pose this question to each group:

"How much of what you have proposed would, in reality, be challenged or not acceptable to your agency?"

Module Six	Services Users and Carers

Potential Training Exercise: "What if......?" A guided fantasy

PURPOSE/OBJECTIVE

To invite participants to reflect on what feelings and reactions might be present if a close relative were to be diagnosed as having a serious mental health difficulty. If you were a user or carer......?

MATERIALS (Optional)

1. A copy of the questions/signposts/images to be used by the trainer in guiding the exercise. [See overleaf]
2. A relatively quiet, comfortable environment "protected" from interruptions/telephone calls/outside noise!

PROCESS

1. The trainer describes personal nature of exercise, checking acceptability, consent, objectives.

2. The participants are encouraged to find comfortable "space" in which to reflect anywhere in the room and to do whatever they usually do when wanting to relax, yet be receptive.

3. When everyone is settled, invite the participants to picture in their minds a beginning scenario as described below.

4. Pose a series of questions/signposts with time to consider responses.

5. When completed, suggest that the participants talk in pairs (with someone they know or feel comfortable with) about the feelings that they experienced as the fantasy progressed.

6. Brief plenary to see how participants feel now. "What has this exercise left you with?", and so on.

THE SCENARIO

Try and imagine a set of circumstances in which you learn that a close relative (mother/father/brother/sister) [CHOOSE ONE] is in hospital following a slight stroke. Further diagnoses indicate that s/he has also signs of senile dementia and the current view is that s/he can no longer live at home without considerable support and care. The options being voiced are either that s/he comes to live with you, or enters residential care.

NOTES FOR TRAINERS AND PARTICIPANTS

1. All "live" exercises of this nature are capable of triggering past or current experiences in a way that may bring some distress, personal disclosures and reactions. This can, therefore, introduce a powerful dynamic into a workshop group or if reflecting alone. This dynamic must be respected.

2. Debriefing, and allowing sufficient time for participants to acknowledge any impact from the exercise is important. It is likely that "echoes" from this session will be heard in subsequent discussion/reflection.

3. Timing. It is suggested that this exercise is only introduced to a workshop when participants have established some degree of comfort and trust with each other and the trainers.

QUESTIONS / SIGNPOSTS

1. What is the first thing that enters your mind?

2. How do/would you feel about these options?

3. How easy/difficult/possible would it be to accommodate him/her in practical housing/ economic terms?

4. How would s/he feel about the prospect of coming to live with you?

5. What would be the impact on your life, and others in the family, for example, your own children, your partner, and so on........? (In financial, physical, emotional, social terms etc)

6. What would you have to change to make it possible?

7. How do you feel now?

● ●

This module - "Sample Training Exercises" - is one of 7 modules in "Learning Materials on Mental Health - An Introduction" . The other modules include:

Module 1 - "Recognition of Mental Health Problems"
Module 2 - "Intervention and Management"
Module 3 - "Legislation and Guidance"
Module 4 - "Special Client Groups"
Module 5 - "Special Issues"
Module 6 - "Users, Carers and Children of Parents with Mental Health Problems"

A sister set of materials is also available for professionals involved in assessing risk - "Learning Materials on Mental Health Risk Assessment"

trainer's appendix

SOME KEY POINTS &
CASE STUDIES

Positive Symptoms of Schizophrenia

Hallucinations
Auditory

Visual

Somatic (touch)

of taste (Gustatory)

of smell (Olfactory)

Delusions
Paranoid

Grandiose

of Reference

Interference with control of behaviour & thinking
Passivity

Thought broadcasting

Thought insertion and

withdrawal

Negative Symptoms of Schizophrenia

Lack of energy and drive

Lack of interest

Poverty of thought

Lack of social interaction

Loss of feelings and emotion

Slowness of thought and movement

CASE STUDY: Barry

Barry Horton is 25 years old and lives with his middle-aged-parents.

Last year, Barry began to become more and more withdrawn and his parents felt he was "strange". When they spoke to him, he did not reply properly, stared a lot, and seemed preoccupied with an inner world, often "talking to himself". One night he cut up several items of clothing and threw them out of his bedroom window. He then became "explosive", shouting and running outside for no clear reason. He said that voices told him he was smelling of urine, and he couldn't prove them wrong because "they come from another atmosphere".

Barry was hospitalised twice in the following year and treated with antipsychotic medication. This had the effect of treating his hallucinations and other psychotic symptons, but he now appears to be lethargic and lacking in drive, and communicates in a monotone. He is also usually restless and paces around much of the time with seeming little purpose.

CASE STUDY: Pauline

Pauline is 32 years old and has 3 children aged 10, 7 and 2 years old. Pauline was treated for depression after the births of the two youngest children, and the death of her mother.

A year ago Jack, Pauline's husband, left the family home after an affair with a younger woman. In the month following this, Pauline became increasingly depressed and began smoking heavily. Standards of household care deteriorated rapidly and the two oldest children were often absent from school. Pauline felt that the future was empty and hopeless. She described herself as a "bad mother" and felt that she had nothing to give to her children. She was tired and listless, unable to sleep. She lost weight as she often felt that she could not face her food.

Last month, Pauline was admitted to hospital after taking an overdose. She was discharged after two weeks and is currently being treated with anti depressants. Her mother-in-law is helping her care for the children.

CASE STUDY: Dorothy

Dorothy is 50 years old, and has been divorced for 11 years. She lives with her mother who is in good health, and her student daughter. Dorothy is outgoing and "chatty" as a personality, and has many friends through her work as a receptionist for a large engineering company.

In recent weeks, Dorothy is described as having become unusually "moody", weeping at times, but rapidly recovering. In the past 2-3 days she has become excitable and has developed an enormous drive to redecorate and furnish the whole house. She ordered 300 metres of curtain material at an expensive store, and stayed up for three nights making curtains. When they were finished she declared them "not good enough" and ordered even more expensive fabric to replace them. To pay for it, she wrote cheques for enormous amounts, which the bank refused to honour. At work there have been episodes of unusual explosions of anger, and excitable, rapid and over-familiar conversations with business clients.

12 months on

In her first period of illness, Dorothy was admitted to hospital under the *Mental Health Act, 1983,* and treated with neuroleptic drugs. She recovered and returned to work, but has had two similar episodes since, which were highly disruptive of her family life. Following the second she lost her job. Her mother has become anxious and weary and is unable to sleep. She is being treated for raised blood pressure. She says she feels she is on a permanent "knife edge", and is terrified by the way Dorothy loses of control when she is ill.

CASE STUDY: Mr Lee

Mr. Lee is 79 years of age and lives at home with his wife. He retired from his career as a senior executive within a retail business at the age of 65 and has since enjoyed a healthy retirement.

Over the last year or so, however, Mr. Lees' golfing friends have noticed that "his memory appears to be failing him". Previously Mr. Lee had never failed to miss an arranged game, but over the past few months he has missed several due to his forgetfulness. At home his wife feels that Mr. Lee is becoming increasingly confused. Sometimes he appears to forget where he is, at other times he cannot remember the names of members of his family and his friends.

More recently, Mr. Lee appears to be showing little interest in his appearance. His wife now has to remind him to take a bath and comb his hair. Mrs. Lee regards this as a sign that "something just isn't right. He's always looked so well turned-out. I've never seen him neglect himself like this before".

Last week Mrs. Lee discussed the situation with her sons. They too felt that there had been a gradual change in Mr. Lee's behaviour and appearance over the past two years and suggested that Mrs. Lee should ask the GP to visit.

CASE STUDY: Carly

Carly is 26 years old and is a lone parent of four children aged 8 years, 7 years, 3 years and 21 months.

Carly spent much of her early life in care, following physical and suspected sexual abuse by her step-father. Carly lived in a number of different children's homes and foster homes, and the records reveal a pattern of increasingly problematic behaviour.

In her early teens, Carly began running away and missing school. She was placed on probation for setting fire to a school when she was 15yrs old. Carly became pregnant at 17 years of age, and married her boyfriend (who also had a care history). They had two children, but then parted following the husband's imprisonment following a robbery.

Carly has since had several relationships with men, and is unsure who the father of her fourth child is.

Carly continues to be the concern of many agencies. Her children are all on the Child Protection Register, due to incidents when Carly had left them alone overnight. The two youngest have had hospital admissions following domestic accidents. Carly denies any difficulties with the children and says that neighbours and friends are to blame for "letting her down".

Carly has harmed herself on several occasions in moments of crisis, and has been admitted twice to a psychiatric unit on a section of the *Mental Health Act, 1983,* however, these incidents become meaningless to her once the crisis is over.

Carly is subject to a probation order for fraud and illegal reconnection of a meter.

Carly has poor relationships with family and friends, and her relationships with professionals are fraught. She perceives people as being "for or against her", and cannot tolerate any challenge. She refuses to talk to social workers since the children were put on the Child Protection Register. She makes excessive demands on other professionals for support.

Because of escalating concerns about the welfare and development of the four children, it is likely that the children will be removed into the care of the local authority under an order of the *Children Act, 1989.* Her housing tenure is also in jeopardy because of rent debt, and complaints from neighbours about the behaviour of visitors to the home.

FROM MODULE 1

Case example of the Supervision Register: James

James Holland (28 years) was admitted to hospital informally, experiencing acute psychotic symptoms, later diagnosed as schizophrenia. He said that he was chosen by God to fight off evil spirits, and he had set fire to his home as part of this delusion. His wife was terrified as she had not experienced him behaving in this way before. He had become abusive to her, and she said she wanted an immediate divorce.

Mr. Holland recovered from the acute illness in about three weeks, and was able to talk to his wife, but did not acknowledge that he had been ill at all. The only precipitating factor in his illness appeared to be the loss of his job some months previously and a growing loss of confidence in his value to an employer.

Mrs. Holland told the psychiatrist that she was prepared to have her husband back but was afraid that it would happen again, particularly as he was not acknowledging any problem. Mr. Holland did not see the need for any support on discharge, although he responded well to staff generally. He felt that medication was unnecessary.

At a CPA meeting, it was felt that some support and monitoring of the situation would be important in view of the fire-setting (which could have killed both of them) and Mrs.Holland's fears. It was decided that the risk justified placing Mr.Holland's name on the Supervision Register and a social worker was allocated to the case. Mr.Holland was not happy with being put on the Register, but got on well with the social worker and accepted help in finding further educational opportunities. Mrs. Holland asked for information and explanations about schizophrenia which seemed to help her. She felt that without the Supervision Register, her husband would probably not accept the social worker's visits. Regular out-patient appointments were arranged to monitor Mr.Holland's progress without medication.

The Care Programme Approach, Circular HC(90)23/LASSL(90)11, 1990.

- Systematic assessment of the health and social care needs of psychiatric patients, particularly where there is a severe and enduring mental illness.

- Drawing up a "package of care" agreed with members of the multi-disciplinary team, local authority care managers, GPs, service users and their carers.

- Nomination of a key worker, who will keep close contact with the client and carers, or family.

- Regular review and monitoring of the client's needs and progress, and of the delivery of the care programme.

Disorders of Childhood

- **Emotional disorders** - anxiety, phobias, mild depression, obsessive compulsive disorder.

- **Conduct Disorders** - non-compliant oppositional behaviour, stealing, fire-setting, aggression, substance abuse.

- **Hyperactive Disorders** - attention deficit hyperactive disorder.

- **Developmental Disorders** - either specific, for example, in speech and language, or pervasive, for example, autism.

- **Eating Disorders** - anorexia nervosa, bulimia.

- **Psychotic Disorders** - schizophrenia, major depression, mania.

- **Somatic Disorders** - chronic fatigue syndrome.

WHICH FACTORS MAY INCREASE THE RISK OF VIOLENCE IN MENTALLY ILL PEOPLE?

These risk factors appear to be linked with an increased risk of violence to others:

- history of violent behaviour;

- high levels of anger/hostility;

- clinical diagnosis (including personality disorders, manic depression and schizophrenia);

- active symptoms (particularly delusions and hallucinations);

- medication non compliance and/or failing to attend appointments;

- concurrent substance abuse;

- homelessness;

- presence of situational factors, particularly those that have been associated with past violence and in particular the first offence

CHILDREN'S NEEDS

In assessing whether the needs of children are being met, the following areas should be considered:

- Does a parent (or adult in a parental role) generally anticipate the child's needs for food, clothing, sleep, play and safety?

- Does a parent respond to the child's initiatives, offer warm interactions, and respond to distress?

- Does a parent refer to the child positively, or describe them with warmth?

- Does a parent set reasonably age-appropriate boundaries to the child's behaviour?

- Does the parent expect to "look after" the child, rather than the child being expected to "look after" the parent?

- Does a parent offer a consistent and continuing relationship with the child, over time?

- Are any periods of separation managed reasonably in relation to the age of the child?

- As the child develops, is he or she supported in relationships with the world outside of the immediate household?

- Is the child free from abuse?

GLOSSARY OF ABBREVIATIONS USED

ASW
Approved Social Worker

CPA
Care Programme Approach

CPN
Community Psychiatric Nurse

CMHT
Community Mental Health Team

DSM-IV & ICD-10
Two systems used in diagnosing mental illness

DV
Domiciliary Visit

ECT
Electro-Convulsive Therapy

EE
Expressed Emotion

EPA
Enduring Power of Attorney

FSW
Family Support Worker

GAD
Generalised Anxiety Disorder

GP
General Practitioner

HSG
Health Service Guidance

IQ
Intelligence Quotient (a system for measuring intelligence)

MID
Multi-Infarct Dementia

MISG
Mental Illness Specific Grant

NHS
National Health Service

OCD
Obsessive-Compulsive Disorder

PD
Personality Disorder

SSRI
Serotonin Specific Reuptake Inhibitor (a type of antidepressant)

MENTAL HEALTH CARE ORGANISATIONS

Listed below are the details of a number of mental health organisations in the United Kingdom - please note that this list is by no means exhaustive.

Alcoholics Anonymous
PO Box 1
Stonebow House
Stonebow
York YO1 2NJ
(01904) 644026

CRUSE Bereavement Care
Cruse House,
126 Sheen Road
Richmond
Surrey TW9 1UR
(0181) 940 4818

Depressives Anonymous
36 Chestnut Avenue
Beverley
East Yorkshire HU17 9QU
(01482) 860619

Good Practices in Mental Health
380-384 Harrow Road
London W9 2HU
(0171) 289 2034

Making Space
46 Allen Street
Warrington
Cheshire WA2 7JB
(01925) 571680

Manic Depression Fellowship Ltd
8-10 High Street
Kingston-on-Thames
Surrey KT1 1EY
(0181) 974 6550

Mental Health Foundation
37 Mortimer Street
London W1N 8JU
(0171) 580 0145

MIND
Granta House
15-19 Broadway
Stratford
London E15 4BQ
(0181) 519 2122

National Schizophrenia Fellowship
28 Castle Street
Kingston-Upon Thames
Surrey KT1 1SS
(0181) 547 3937

Phobics Society
4 Cheltenham Road
Manchester M21 1QN
(0161) 881 1937

Relate National Marriage Guidance
Herbert Gray College,
Little Church Street,
Rugby,
Warwickshire CV21 3AP
(01788) 573241

Sainsbury Centre for Mental Health
134-138, Borough High Street,
London SE1 1LB
(0171) 403 8790

Survivors Speak Out
34 Osnaburgh Street
London NW1 3ND
(0171) 916 5472/3

The Carers National Association
20-25 Glasshouse Yard,
London EC1A 4JF

The Mental Health After Care Association
25 Bedford Square
London WC1B 3HW
(0171) 436 6194

The Samaritans
10 The Grove
Slough
Berkshire SL1 1QP
(01753) 532713

Turning Point
101 Backchurch Lane
London E1 1LU
(0171) 702 2300

UK Advocacy Group
Premier House
14 Cross Burgess Street
Sheffield S1 2HG
(0114) 275 3131